She's Tough
Extreme Fitness Training for Women

Kylie Hatmaker and Mark Hatmaker

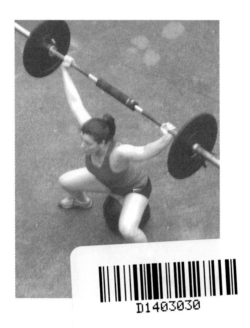

D1403030

Cover and interior photos by Doug Werner

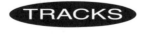

Tracks Publishing
San Diego, California

She's Tough
Extreme Fitness Training for Women
Kylie Hatmaker and Mark Hatmaker

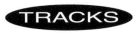

Tracks Publishing
140 Brightwood Avenue
Chula Vista, CA 91910
619-476-7125
tracks@cox.net
www.startupsports.com
trackspublishing.com

Copyright © 2014 by Kylie Hatmaker, Mark Hatmaker and Doug Werner
10 9 8 7 6 5 4 3 2 1

Publisher's Cataloging-in-Publication

Hatmaker, Kylie.

She's tough : extreme fitness training for women / Kylie Hatmaker and Mark Hatmaker ; cover and interior photos by Doug Werner. -- San Diego, California : Tracks Publishing, c2014.

p. ; cm.

ISBN: 978-1-935937-61-6
Includes index.
Summary: There is a growing interest among a niche of active women to engage in extreme sporting activities that require the highest level of conditioning. High Intensity Training (HIT) addresses that and this book addresses that specifically for women. Featured are scores of core exercises illustrated in action sequence, along with chapters on what is possible and what is not, eating and training, grooming, training partners, and building a home gym.--Publisher.

1. Physical fitness for women. 2. Exercise for women. 3. Weight training for women. 4. Women--Health and hygiene. 5. Extreme sports--Training. I. Hatmaker, Mark. II. Werner, Doug, 1950- III. Title.

GV439 .H38 2014   2014936463
613.7/045--dc23   1407

Books by Mark Hatmaker

No Holds Barred Fighting:
The Ultimate Guide to Submission Wrestling

More No Holds Barred Fighting:
Killer Submissions

No Holds Barred Fighting:
Savage Strikes

No Holds Barred Fighting:
Takedowns

No Holds Barred Fighting:
The Clinch

No Holds Barred Fighting:
The Ultimate Guide to Conditioning

No Holds Barred Fighting:
The Kicking Bible

No Holds Barred Fighting:
The Book of Essential Submissions

Boxing Mastery

No Second Chance:
A Reality-Based Guide to Self-Defense

MMA Mastery:
Flow Chain Drilling and Integrated O/D Training

MMA Mastery:
Ground and Pound

MMA Mastery:
Strike Combinations

Boxer's Book of Conditioning & Drilling

Boxer's Bible of Counterpunching

Mud, Guts & Glory
Tips & Training for Extreme Obstacle Racing

Books are available through major bookstores
and booksellers on the Internet.

This book is dedicated to
two recently departed
grandparents.

Ernestine "Ernie" Barrs.
In a good movie or a
good book happy endings
are paramount — she
topped them all.

And to Roy Kenneth
"Nubbin" Tucker, on
whom I can bestow his
ultimate compliment —
he was a good man.

It is an honor to be
descended from both of
them.

Acknowledgments
Phyllis Carter
Editor Extraordinaire

Contents

Introduction: *Let's Talk*

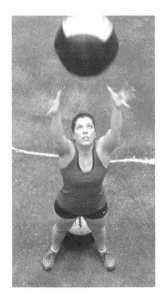

Welcome to my book!

I'm going to level with you — I've never written a book before so if you meet up with a few areas where you think to yourself, "Wow, that was a little rough" I hope you'll cut me some slack.

I'm not coming at this without some help. First of all my husband, Mark, has written beaucoup books and was with me all the way. You will see them listed in this very guide.

I had even more help in the person of the publisher of this book, Doug Werner. He has written many a book himself, and I count him as a friend. So I'm not alone in this endeavor — I've got a couple of old hands looking over my shoulder.

The piece of advice that really stuck with me was "Forget about writing a book, instead, talk the book." That is, make the book a conversation between me, the author, and you, the reader. I really liked that and I think it worked.

That's exactly what I'll be doing throughout — talking to you as if you and I were together in the same room or the same gym or on the same running trail discussing the subject in question: Women getting fit — you and I getting seriously fit without sacrificing our femininity.

So, let's start the conversation ...

Hi, my name is, Kylie. Welcome to my book. I hope you learn something along the way.

I know I did.

I'm chugging at the atmosphere like a drowning swimmer going under for the last time.

1.1 *Heart Attack Hill*

So here's how it all started ...

Our driveway sits on a hill. It's approximately 100 yards long with a somewhat steep portion as you near the top. Keep that 100 yards in mind. I'm not talking a mile, just an upward sloping football field.

About five years ago my husband, step-daughter, Samantha, and I were riding our bikes on the nice level area down near the house. We didn't do this often, but for some reason something about that afternoon prompted a little "Hey, we're a family riding our bikes in circles" action.

After a few short flat laps Mark got bored, headed up the hill, hit the top and then shot back down to grab that joyful bit of effortless speed that only going downhill on a bike can give.

He's doing this over and over and soon Samantha gets into the up-the-hill-slowly, down-the-hill-quickly action.

> ## "What the hell just happened to me?"

Me? I'm content with the flat lazy circles we started with down below. But after a few prompts of "Come on, it's fun" and not wanting to be the party-pooper in the impromptu family bike party, I attacked the hill.

Remember what I said about 100 yards? Let's break that 100 yards down into increments.

First 25-30 yards. Piece of cake, should have joined them in the fun earlier.

30-50 yards. Hmm? A little steeper than I thought, but I'm fine.

50-75 yards. I am peddling through molasses. Moving so slowly that I wonder how I can have enough forward momentum to keep the bike upright. Also, how is a 10-year-old going up and down this hill with no problem? I might have to ground her.

75 to 90 yards. Nobody knows it but I am seriously contemplating quitting. I'm 10 yards from the top of the hill, standing up on the pedals and driving for all I'm worth and making what seems to my oxygen depleted lungs like zero progress.

Top of the Hill. I do not hairpin turn and hit the down-hill immediately as my two now-hated family members do. I stop, put both feet on the pavement and huff for breath hoping that my discomfort is not as obvious as I fear it must be.

I'm taking short ragged breaths at an alarming clip. This is 100 yards people, and I'm chugging at the atmosphere like a drowning swimmer going under for the last time.

My heart! I don't think I've ever been so acutely aware of it before. It's pounding so hard and rapidly I think, "My God, I'm 28-years-old, lean with no pre-existing health problems and I'm going to keel over in my own driveway, felled by what is essentially a child's toy."

I eventually regained some semblance of normal breathing and rode down the hill. It was not as fun as they said. Perhaps because I was too busy doing the internal mental assessment of "What the hell just happened to me?" to appreciate the wind-in-the-face moment.

At the bottom, I continued the lazy flat circles, left the hill to them and thought to myself, "Whoa, I am one seriously out-of-shape loser."

Note to reader: Being out of shape didn't really make me a loser — remember, I write how I talk. I'm just saying this was a wake-up call. I had a decision to make, I could go one of three ways:

1. Sell the bikes and forbid anyone from ever using them again.

2. Start yoga or Pilates, or some other form of "does this pass for exercise?" to make me feel better about myself while still riding my flat circles and avoiding hills for the rest of my life. Or ...

3. Really do something about what just happened to me.

I think you know which one I chose.

1.2 What's Wrong with Pilates?

Nuthin'.

Yeah, I kinda knocked it there a bit. Well, that and yoga. And if you want to know the truth I put Zumba, Jazzercise and whatever else has been, is, or will be new and trendy and marketed primarily to a female audience in the same weak sauce category.

I personally don't like the assumptions that what all we sweet little ladies need is some tarted up phys ed lite confection that we can all do in a little room isolated from the real gym equipment. Who started this whole women are delicate flowers who are only capable of dancing or stretching their way to fitness while wearing marketed-just-for-the-class trendy clothes?

Talk about gender stereotypes — there you have 'em.

Listen — if any of the above are your personal cups of (weak) tea, knock yourself out, I'm not here to talk anyone out of their tea.

> ## Some of us want to be challenged, not "empowered." I hate that word, it smacks of condescension.

I'm simply saying that some of us prefer coffee. You know, something a little stronger. Something that will get the job done right now.

Some of us want to be challenged, not "empowered." I hate that word, it smacks of condescension. I've never understood the self-imposed contradiction of "I'm equal to any man and when I get through with my step class with my five pound hand weights I'll prove it."

This book, as if you didn't already know, is aimed at those women who already resent this condescension. Or who at the very least suspect that some of the "Just for Ladies" fitness regimes might be lacking.

Again, if you like the tea, drink all of it you like, just never forget it's weak tea and nothing more.

Me? I like my coffee strong.

I remember when I first started working out. What to me now are the simplest tasks seemed like insurmountable challenges. Each time we tackle something that we find difficult and then overcome that obstacle, or at the very least give it our best shot, we grow a bit better or stronger for simply having attempted to do what was

13

> We improve ourselves by the effort we put in, not the comfort we escape to.

in front of us.

I've learned that we grow not only in physical capacity but in mental capacity. Old-timers used to call it grit. We learn that you make hard tasks easier not by lowering the bar, but by keeping the bar high and always trying to meet and exceed what's in front of you. We improve ourselves by the effort we put in, not the comfort we escape to.

Some may think that always keeping the bar high might create frustration, but I don't see it that way because there is no failure in showing up and doing the work to whatever capacity you are currently capable of. The only failure is not showing up at all, not even attempting the work, or purposefully diminishing the work before we even commence so that a false sense of self-esteem grows as we require less of ourselves.

1.3 No Boys Allowed (Unless ...)

Having training partners, or better yet, an entire crew of people to work with while you're training, working out, whatever you want to call it, can make the whole affair a bit more fun. Having a companion or two sweating, straining and shouting encouragement side-by-side can go a long way to making some of the hard work required a bit more palatable.

In choosing training partners, some go out of their way to stay gender-specific. That is, avoiding a co-ed crew. I see this as a mistake. No, there's nothing wrong with having a female-only crew if only females want to step up. But I do think there is a problem with intentionally creating a female-only crew.

I was all prepared to lay down my thoughts on this when I recalled my husband had already written on this very subject. So I'm going to allow him to highjack the conversation for the next few paragraphs. Keep in mind he is writing to an audience that is interested in Mixed Martial Arts and Combat Training, but it seems to me that, all the thoughts hold true for our conversation.

So, take it away, Hon.

1.4 Gender & Weight Class
by Mark Hatmaker

I am often asked a question along these lines, "Hey Mark, I have some women in my class. What's the best approach to teaching them?"

My answer: "Like a fully functioning, intelligent human being with an interest in combat sports or street defense."

Many gyms offer female-only classes in what seems to me some curious harkening back to "separate but equal" days.

Before anyone running or gladly attending a single-gender mandated class gets his hackles up, stand down. I am completely aware that many women (not all) prefer the female-only approach. When it is the individual's call to be separated from others, by all means exercise that preference.

I'm talking to those who may have wondered why the genders must be separated (I see no reason for it), or, if the genders are mixed, should there be a difference in treatment? (Not so much).

From what I can tell in conversation with many, these questions are way stickier than they appear at first blush. So let's see if we can make things a little less sticky.

First, if you are a female and prefer the company of a female-only crew, that's your call — I'm not here to talk you out of it. I would, however, ask why you prefer working with your gender alone. In asking this question I've received some of the following answers.

"I find working with women less threatening."

OK, that's fair. But no matter your gender, if you find your current coaches or training partners threatening, then maybe they aren't the ones you should train with. The ideal environment to foster learning is one that will challenge you, constantly raise the bar (your per-

> The ideal environment to foster learning is one that will challenge you ... and be hell-bent on encouraging you ... to get to new levels.

sonal bar, that is) and be hell-bent on encouraging you and coaching you to get to new levels. Threats in the fiery college basketball coach sense has no place in the equation.

I would be completely thick-skulled if I did not acknowledge that some women turn to self-defense in response to an unpleasant incident in their real lives. I have encountered two polarizing attitudes in women who have endured such a thing.

One group of ladies say, "Don't candy-coat it, I want the real thing because that is never, ever happening to me again." These ladies are my heroes.

The second group have an attitude that is more withdrawn and less likely to accept the interplay and full scope of training that is vital to inculcate real-world skills.

I sympathize and empathize with both attitudes, but I will say that the more assertive one is far more useful. For those less assertive I offer the following advice: If you have chosen your coaches and training partners

Taking it easy with your female cohort is in a sense saying, "You can't handle this ..."

well, then trust your judgment and get to training. These folks are your partners in the game, they are here to help.

If you do not trust them enough to give yourself up to the training, then get out of there and move on to where you can feel comfortable. If that place is nowhere at the moment, then might I suggest putting training on the back burner for a little while. Give it a little time.

"I don't want to get hurt."

Not getting hurt is a mighty smart stance to take. I am a possessor of male genitalia, and I can testify (note the root of that word) that I don't want to get hurt either. I can't think of a man or woman I have trained with who has approached training sessions with a desire to suffer an injury.

With that said, we must accept the fact that combat training is a contact sport, and there will there be a few bumps and bruises down the line. That is, if you're doing it right. All contact will be scaled to skill and weight class (coming to that), but expecting to absorb the full impact of the training (so to speak) in a hands-off method is akin to expecting to become proficient at football or rugby without allowing for any blocking or tackling.

To be frank, I often find classes where the genders are mixed problematic in the opposite sense — the male partners are often a bit too solicitous of their female counterparts. They are behaving quite the opposite of what some fear, they are being considerate gentlemen. As much as a fan of respect, honor and manners that I am, I find this over-solicitation a disservice to the women.

I'm not saying don't be courteous, don't be a gentleman, but I am saying that this over-extension of "taking it easy" actually implies the opposite of respect (unknowingly and unintentionally, of course). Taking it easy with your female cohort is in a sense saying, "You can't handle this, so I will treat you with kid gloves."

This isn't license to knock your female partners out (if you were capable or even of the inclination). It's just a bit of advice to treat each other as the considerate, intelligent, able human beings that each of you are.

Rather than the sexes avoiding or tip-toeing around one another, I suggest we regard one another as the athletes or burgeoning athletes that we are. If we are going to adjust for differences, let's let those adjustments be in deference to a distinction we already make — weight class.

Contrary to popular myth and in agreement with a particular type of email spam, size matters. Size differences are why we have weight classes. Combat classes are often composed of athletes of all sorts of shapes and sizes, and we are all perfectly used to the idea of holding back a little when you are much bigger than your partner or pushing a little harder when your partner is bigger than you. What I'm saying, guys and gals, play like your weight class, not your gender.

A couple more thoughts on the subject before we sign off here.

Some grappling positions are a little, um, comical to the rookies in a co-ed crowd. These positions may lead some to think, "Oh, how would that look if I did that?"

Answer: It would look like you're training.

To those who sweat the "compromising" grappling positions, it's not merely a gender-mix hesitation. Most same-gender-only participants ponder the same thoughts on their first day. It's fun to tell two beefy Marines to lie down and one get between the others legs. The first time they may cock an eyebrow, but then it all quickly turns to business because that's what it is.

And then there's the tears factor. Men and women possess different ratios of the hormones testosterone and estrogen — and viva la difference! These hormones can cause some (not all) individuals to involuntarily express stress or frustration differently.

In some women, that stress expression is tears. Are these tears signs of weakness?

These tears are no more signs of weakness in women

> ... tears are no more signs of weakness in women than they are in males who cry upon winning inside the octagon.

than they are in males who cry upon winning inside the octagon.

There's a fine scene in the film "Courage Under Fire," which concerns a female chopper pilot performing well in a combat situation. One of the crew derisively observes, "The captain's crying!" The pilot (played by Meg Ryan) says plainly, "It's stress, that's all.

And that's all there is to it. Some men express stress with false braggadocio and some women tear up. Female UFC phenom Rhonda Rousey is said to cry at some point practically every day in her training. Anyone think she's weak?

Nah, me neither.

1.5 False Starts & Excuses a la Carte

OK, back to me.

From that *Heart Attack Hill* story onward, I know I've sounded all nose to the grindstone, do or die, come hell or high water and Mrs. Rock-Solid-Motivation.

Well, it wasn't always that way.

> **Most of us need some sort of kick in the pants to get going ...**

It's not always that way now.

I had numerous false starts before Heart Attack Hill. All of the usual "Hey, I'm gonna get in shape" pronouncements of the New Year's Resolution variety and a few that were sparked by an upcoming swimsuit season. Sometimes my good intentions were simply because I thought it was the right thing to do for my health.

When I took steps in the right direction, most of these were of the "Ladies only" variety that I knocked around a few pages back. So let's be clear, there was a time in my life when I wasn't motivated or disciplined enough to stick with something that I personally didn't find very challenging at all.

Why didn't I stick with it?

Well, you and I know the answer to that one. Doing nothing is way easier than doing something. That's just the truth of it.

The fact that we haven't done something or stuck with something in our lives doesn't mean we suck as human beings, it means we're simply being human beings.

Let's face it. Most of us need some sort of kick in the pants to get going, whether that comes in the form of a bicycle induced cardiac event, that high school reunion around the corner, or an overheard "chunky" comment from a stranger who needs whispering lessons.

Me? I had all the excuses loaded and ready...

"It's mighty cold outside, it can't be healthy to go running in this sort of weather." Used it.

"It's mighty hot outside, it can't be healthy to exercise in this sort of weather." Check.

"I've got to get up early for work tomorrow, I really need my rest." I loved this one.

"I overslept today and really need to catch up." That one, too.

"Aw, I was going to workout tonight but my friend and workout buddy can't make it, so I'll wait for her because we're a team." This one is popular because it makes us sound compassionate and altruistic, but I'll remind you that no matter how often your friend does or does not show up for workout will not change the size and sag of your butt. Nope, your butt is your responsibility.

And on and on.

You sense a pattern? No matter the circumstances a human being can be counted on to come up with a nice sounding rationalization even if the excuses examined in series are contradictory.

My favorites were always of this variety:

"Kylie's Great Big Grand Super-Duper Exercise &
Nutrition Program … (wait for it) starts tomorrow …
or this weekend … or at the first of the month … or as
soon as I have my oil changed … or ….

Yeah, this was my big favorite. Big plans that were
never scheduled to start today, right now. Always
tomorrow, or some other time that ain't right here.

I've found that this is pretty common, the "Oh, out-of-
shape body, just you wait until Thursday and you will
not believe the paces I'm gonna put you through."
Invariably Thursday arrives and it turns into an Orange
is the New Black viewing marathon.

Well, we all need some motivation to get us going and
keep us moving: heart attacks, swim suits, inconsider-
ately shrinking pants, et cetera. Some words of wisdom
to keep in mind to get us over that "Well, I said I was
going to tonight but …" moments.

For some, Nike's "Just do it!" is golden, and there is
something admirable in its sleek wisdom. But those
three words sound like something said by folks who
are already doing what they're doing to we not-doing-it-
yet folks.

You know, easier-said-than-done advice.

Here's one I use, I cribbed it from my husband, who
uses it all the time on himself, first a teensy story to set
it in context.

> **"So, tomorrow you shall be a good man, what does that make you today?"**

The Stoic philosopher, Epictetus, offered this retort to a student who professed grand plans of learning and moral deeds he was planning on starting the next day:

"So, tomorrow you shall be a good man, what does that make you today?"

Ouch!

If we applied this logic to all grand plans in our lives, we can see that unstated opposite in each pronouncement we make:

"Tomorrow I'll start that diet, today I shall be fat."

"I'll train hard starting tomorrow, today I am lazy."

"Tomorrow I'll work toward last year's slacks, today I'll sign up for a Lane Bryant catalog."

So, what are you doing today?

1.6 Texas Proverb

Let's stay hardcore and maintain our all-out assault on the bottomless well of excuses for a few more paragraphs.

First, the Texas Proverb, which was a folk saying among

> **Are we cowards, weaklings, or unfit? And always the answer is, hopefully, none of the above.**

Texas settlers in the early to mid-18th century regarding migration to the newly open Texas Territory:

Cowards Never Started,
The Weak Never Got Here
& the Unfit Don't Stay.

That's some strong medicine. My husband and I were so struck by the grit and determination starkly expressed in those three lines that it is stenciled on a wall in our home so we can ask ourselves each day with whatever we are facing: Are we cowards, weaklings, or unfit? And always the answer is, hopefully, none of the above.

We don't have to be talking about something as daunting as pulling up roots and heading for unknown country full of Comanche, Apache and Mexican Federales who didn't want us there. We can apply this strong medicine to how we approach our training, or about anything in life that is more than a little tough to get going or stick with.

Here's the deal when confronting the Texas Proverb — be honest with yourself about whatever it is you are applying the proverb to.

If you don't want to put the effort in, admit that to

yourself. There's nothing wrong with that. Say I'm comfortable with how I look, how I feel, and never riding a bike up a hill.

I've got no quibble with this kind of personal assessment, it's honest and, as a matter of fact, it is honorable.

This sort of admission is far preferable than any of the countless:

"Oh, I would if my back wasn't so ..."

"If I were younger I would ..."

"If I had more time I would ..."

And on and on and on and on.

Having the guts to say I have no interest in going to Texas (in reality or metaphorically) is simply a statement of preference and has no value judgment attached to it. But ...

Claiming you love Texas and talking about Texas all the time — reading articles and books (this one maybe?) about Texas, but never going; or perhaps packing to go, but stopping short; or getting to Texas and turning around once you realize that it's going to be a little hot — going on about Texas as if it is your destination of choice ... well, that's just fiction.

Quit telling yourself and your friends and your family Texas Tall Tales.

Either decide the journey is worth it and go. Or that Texas ain't in the cards for you.

Don't be the "Well, I would, but …" person. If you are reading this book, I presume our little metaphorical Texas holds some appeal for you. And if so, you may want to ask yourself those three questions each day:

> *Am I a coward?*
> *Am I a weakling?*
> *Am I unfit?*

1.7 Tough Texans of All Types

Starting to think I'm too mean, too tough with all of this "Just shut up and do it" talk?

Hold your horses and let's remind ourselves that it took all sorts to get to Texas. It wasn't just big strong strapping pioneer types. There were school marms and mothers and widows and more than a few babies along for the ride.

I bring this up because the tough talk we are talking about is all relative and scalable to who we are right now; what we're able and capable of doing right now — today at this very moment.

Don't compare yourself with what you wish you could do if you had put the time in by starting earlier. Until Google invents a time machine we're stuck where we are right now with the choices we've made up to this moment.

> **... the tough talk ... is all relative and scalable to who we are right now ... today at this very moment.**

Don't compare yourself unfavorably to someone who has put the time in. They are where they are because they started on the journey to Texas sooner than you, that's all.

Oh, and by the way, don't look at those further on the journey than you and say things like "Well, I could too if ..." Anyone who gets anywhere got there because they put the time and effort in. Any disparaging comment about those already on the journey says more about the disparager than the disparagee.

I mentioned earlier that we get to where we are going not by lowering the bar but by keeping the bar high and always striving for the horizon.

Day One after Heart Attack Hill, I went to work on my metaphorical Texas. I had never done a pull-up in my life. Never. Not one pull-up in 28 years on the planet.

I go to that pull-up bar, I grip it and struggle for all I'm worth, and guess what?

Barely budged. I'm basically hanging at full arm's extension at the bottom of the bar wriggling like a fish on a hook and my, oh-so-supportive husband is cackling with practically wet-your-pants glee.

> **It took me a good six months to get that chin over the bar for the first time for one measly rep.**

I come off the bar and say, "I can't do this."

He says, "Of course you can't. You've never worked at it before. Babies can't walk from day one, they have to practice."

In other words, you have to keep trying, keep wiggling, keep falling down a lot. Not getting the chin over the bar is never failure, any more than it is failure when a toddler takes more than a few months to get this one foot in front of the other thing down pat.

I got back on the bar and every single instance of hardcore, honest wiggling "counted" as a pull-up repetition.

Flash forward 30 days. Guess how many pull-ups I could do?

Zero, if you're counting chin above the bar, but if you're counting slightly higher hilarious wriggles, well, I was that much closer to Texas.

Flash forward 90 days. Guess how many pull-ups?

Still zero. Better wiggles though.

It took me six months to get that chin over the bar for the first time for one measly rep. That's right, you heard me, half a year for one rep, but … I earned it. That was a big day in the Texas journey.

Flash forward to today: How many pull-ups?

Multiple reps and on some days with a good bit of weight strapped to a weight vest to make what was formerly an exercise in futility a brand new challenge.

You see, what I'm getting at is this — it's OK to not be good at stuff. In fact it's more than OK. It's to be expected. Nobody is good at anything they haven't worked at.

It's OK to take a while to get to where you're going as there's no wagon train shortcut to Texas.

You've got to put the long dusty tough miles in. But that's what makes it worth it.

Every wee victory in a tough journey is something to celebrate.

So kudos to you and your wiggling on the pull-up bar moments.

Three cheers for the ridiculously feeble efforts we may initially put in with weights.

High five to your first few months of "You call that a fast pace?" run times.

Every bit of effort you put in gets you one step closer to the Lone Star State. And the Lone Star we're talking about is Y-O-U — with the starring lead role in this little journey to a better, leaner, stronger, tougher state of fitness.

Not everyone who started for Texas was tough from the get-go, but those who stayed with it wound up that way all the same.

1.8 A Period Ends a Sentence. Not Life

One more bit of tough-love and we'll move on to kinder, gentler words. Let's not allow that little quirk of female biology called menstruation put a kink in our plans. Yes, it is an inconvenience (and at times a cramping inconvenience) that our male counterparts don't have to put up with, but let's not allow what is a natural part of our lives to become a "Get Out of Jail Free" card to skip on what we claim we want to do.

Menstruation is a part of us, part of who we are as women. It is not a disease, it is not an illness, it is not a crutch, it is not an excuse to parade as a temporary flag of surrender that allows us to take what is essentially a 12-week per year excuse vacation.

Yes, it can be inconvenient and, yes, there can be cramps and, yes, there can be headaches, but in my experience I have found that the mere act of working out acts as a sort of analgesic and relieves the cramps — most of the time. Sometimes not so much, but that's life.

> Not everyone who started for Texas was tough from the get-go, but those who stayed with it wound up that way all the same.

I've compared my experience with other women who do the work without excuses and they say the same thing — doing the job helps with what comes along with menstruation far more than not doing the job at all.

What I have just said should be encouraging news for all of us, but somewhere out there there are a tentative few who will want to play the "Oh, well, my cramps are different. My menstruation is oh, so impressive that I couldn't possibly …" Blah-blah-blah.

Again, get off the wagon train and stay home.

Female athletes, serious professional or amateur, don't cease their lives for one week every month.

The brave women who now voluntarily go to combat zones as part of our armed forces don't say, "No shooting this week."

Those Texas women a couple of centuries ago did not say, "Pull this wagon over and fend for yourselves, kids, Mama's out for a week."

> **Female athletes, serious professional or amateur, don't cease their lives for one week every month.**

Any time I encounter a woman who wants to argue, "Well, I couldn't possibly do this because…" I often don't even know what to say.

Ladies, I'm on your side. I'm telling you what you can do and what you're capable of. I'm telling you that you're stronger and able to deal with far more than you give yourselves credit for.

I find it baffling. Here I am on their side arguing that they are tough and awesome and some take the paradoxical self-denigrating position of "No, I'm not. Don't you dare call me strong. I'm weak, moody and subject to the whims of biology and I won't have any one tell me that I'm better than that."

Weird, huh?

OK, don't wanna take my word that you're stronger than you give yourself credit for?

Stronger every week of the year and not just 40 of them?
Want a little scientific background on why PMS might best be redescribed as BS?

Below are a couple of reference books for you, both

written by women, women who know what they're talking about. If you want to keep arguing that you're a weakling, take it up with them.

Me? I know you're stronger than you think you are. I'm on your side.

The Mismeasure of Woman
Why women are not the better sex, the inferior sex, or the opposite sex
Carol Tavris, Ph. D.
Don't let that subtitle scare you, her myth busting is truthful and as we all know the truth will set you free.

Spin Sisters
How the Women of the Media Sell Unhappiness and Liberalism to the Women of America
Myrna Blyth
Skip the worries about the political nature of the book, Blyth is a former editor at *Ladies Home Journal* and her inside look at how women have been sold a false bill of goods to make themselves think less of themselves is an infuriating eye-opener.

In a nutshell, there's more money in selling us solutions to fake problems than letting us in on the secret that we're stronger and better than we think.

1.9 21st Century Tough Chicks and How You — Yeah, _You_ — Can Be One of Them

OK, ladies, enough with the "step-up" talk. I assume that if you've made it this far we're on the same page — literally and figuratively.

There has never been a better time for we women who want a little more than Zumba and step class to strut our stuff and test our mettle. Hardcore exercise regimens such as CrossFit, p90x and others count an equal number of men and women in their ranks. Men and women of all age ranges as a matter of fact.

Hardcore co-ed conditioning is so mainstream now that the CrossFit games are broadcast on ESPN, both the men and women's divisions. And these divisions include Masters Divisions, which are geared toward athletes in the following age ranges: 40-44, 45-49, 50-54, 55-59, and 60 plus.

I mention the Masters Division because if anyone out there is wondering, "Am I too old for this?" Nah, you're never too old to do something.

Within these same competitions you will find, in addition to the individual Men's and Women's events, Team Events and some of these events are co-ed teams (3 men/3 women).

Not enough proof that this is the Golden Age of Tough Women?

> **There has never been a better time for we women who want a little more than Zumba and step class to strut our stuff and test our mettle.**

Take a look at the stats on those who compete in your innumerable local 5K runs, half marathons and marathons. Again, you'll find a 50/50 split of male and female athletes.

Want more proof of this being our century, ladies?

Mud runs, adventure runs and obstacle course races have taken the world by storm in the last few years and even here in such events as The Spartan Race, the Tough Mudder, the Warrior Dash, the Rugged Maniac and many others you will find that same 50/50 gender ratio.

Want even more?

The UFC, the world's premier professional mixed martial arts (MMA) franchise in the world's fastest growing sport added a women's division in 2012. This division is not some marketing trick stacked with ringers to lure the curious to some foxy boxing sideshow. It is a division full of seriously talented fighters who happen to be female, who occasionally play the main card. I want you to stop and think about what this means.

The 21st century has seen a new cadre of women of all ages, all levels of conditioning, all walks of life step up and strut their bad selves.

Can you remember a time prior to the first decade of the 21st century when we saw so much equality of gender distribution in what are universally regarded as some pretty tough sports?

Can you imagine your mother, let alone your grandmother, having competed in such events if these same opportunities were available to them? If they were available, do you think we'd see this same ratio of women out there rivaling the boys?

Probably not. Not because our Moms and Grandmas weren't tough or capable — the forbears of these ladies have all made their Texas journeys that were far harder I wager than any of the sports we now play.

I say probably not partially because it was simply not socially acceptable.

When physical conditioning/exercise/physical culture, whatever you want to call it was being rediscovered at the turn of the 19th and 20th centuries, it was almost exclusively a male-dominated arena. Yes, there were and always have been female pioneers in physical conditioning and sports, but these ladies were always more the exception than the rule.

For many, it was considered unladylike for a woman to sweat or to exert herself as a man does.

Even when women were encouraged to be "active" we must never forget that women were, despite extensive evidence to the contrary, considered the "fairer" sex — the weaker sex. With our "shortcomings" in mind the vast majority of women's fitness options were dainty forerunners of today's subpar dance choreography regimens or pretend kickboxing where our toughest opponent is the thin air in front of our lycra encased "fragile" bodies.

I surmise that the long slow journey from "women should not exercise" to "ladies only" fitness to "oh, you guys are just as tough" is simply a remnant of gender bias. It's just culture catching up to reality and leaving discrimination behind.

What's a shame about that gender bias is that so much of it in the last 25 years has been self-imposed. It has been women advising other women to pretend to be a chorus girl or to pretend that that flick of the hand is a punch and that cushioning your conditioning is making any significant inroads to serious physical progress.

The 21st century has seen a new cadre of women of all ages, all levels of conditioning, all walks of life step up and strut their bad selves. I, for one, think that our Moms, our Grandmothers, our Great Grandmothers and all of our Great Greats back to Texas and beyond would be proud of where we are now, where we're going, and what we've left behind.

I know this is a book and it should be all about the written word and the captured images, but ... go ahead and have a look at some of the bad-ass girls I'm talking about.

Google CrossFit Games and have a look at the women's divisions. While you're there, don't forget to have a look at some of the bad girls in the female Masters Division.

Also go to SpartanRace.com and have a look at the video of muddy women (and men) hanging tough.

Also, Google Ronda Rousey, Liz Carmouche, Alexis Davis, Sarah Kaufman, Julie Kedzie, Meisha Tate, Cat Zingano and other such ladies of the UFC and see if your stereotypes of what women who fight are supposed to look like get shattered.

Seriously, do it, right now. Google all of these ladies, get yourself an eyeful and see what tough femininity looks like.

Did you do it?

I'll pretend that's a yes.

Now you know what sort of results I'm selling you in these pages.

> Women working out don't start looking like men any more than men who don't work out start looking like women ...

1.10 This All Sounds Good, But Won't I Get Big Like a Man?

If the preceding phrase is rattling around in your skull or if you've got images of bulky, quasi-hermaphroditic-appearing women from the ranks of female professional bodybuilding burned into your mind, this tells me that you didn't go have a look at the ladies I just asked you to look at.

Did any of them look even vaguely like men to you?

You saw strength …

You saw a bit of muscular definition in some…

But what you didn't see is any female form that could be mistaken for a man from certain angles.

I get that worry. Who wants to get tough if it means we have to give up looking like who we are to get there?

41

> To get the hardcore results we're touting ... takes less time than most standardized exercise sessions.

You won't. We naturally go to these images of steroid-juiced women because for the longest time that has been the other end of the women's fitness extreme that has been fed to us.

On one end we have the cushy advice that holding a couple of 5 pound dumbbells in our hands and taking a brisk walk around our neighborhood is going to make us into Jennifer Aniston. At the other end of the extreme we have anabolic steroid using women who build physiques most men would envy (and not envy in the way we want).

The truth of the matter lies in the middle. We can work H-A-R-D and never ever approach looking like a man.

Do you know why?

Because we're not men. We simply lack the male hormonal cocktail to make us into men. Women working out don't start looking like men any more than men who don't work out start looking like women, they simply look like out of shape men. And women who don't work out look like ... well, out of shape women.

Female bodybuilders get their physiques via hard, hard work and copious amounts of pharmaceuticals to tell their body chemistry to behave a bit more like a man's. That's why you see what you see there.

That's the science. No drugs, no man-like characteristics. So please don't allow this worry to become your excuse. It just ain't gonna happen.

And again, any time you start to worry, pull up those images I asked you to Google earlier — fit men look like fit men and fit women look like fit women.

Nice how Mother Nature made it work out like that, huh?

1.11 Yeah, But ...

Now that we've plowed through the personal backstory, the motivational section and had a look at a few role models living and doing exactly what we have in mind for ourselves, we're getting mighty close to particulars.

Let's knock out some of these with a little Q & A.

"I like what I'm hearing about tough, but won't this take a lot of time? It's not like I have 26 hours in a day, you know?"

I hear you. The time crunch is a common lament and is actually one of the more common reasons why some say they will forgo the tough track and opt for the hour-long Zumba, spin or step-class session instead.

But lament no more my tough sisters, To get the hard-core results we're touting in this book takes less time than most standardized exercise sessions.

"How much less time?"

Well, often your tough session will take even less time than it does for your less-tough friend to drive to her Zumba session.

In other words, you can get tough and be tough and get on with what's next in the day before your yoga counterpart's designer gym bag hits the "exercise" floor.

Doesn't seem possible does it? To show you I'm not just blowing smoke, I will direct you to a few different scientific sources at the end of this section, but if you want to skip what the long-winded folks in lab coats have to say, here it is in a nutshell.

In trial after trial, participants have been broken into three groups.

As a rule Group One is your control. They are assigned no exercise regimen at all during the trial run.

Group Two is assigned what we have been fed to believe for years about long slow distance (LSD) training. That is, getting your heart rate up to a moderate level and sustaining this elevated rate for a specified time — anywhere from 30-60 minutes depending on which "expert" you want to believe that day.

> ... more often than not in test after test ... HIT [high intensity training] exceeds the benefits of LSD [long slow distance] training by a long shot.

Group Three is assigned the new way (the tough way) which is a series of high intensity training intervals (HIT). That is, if Group Two is expected to jog at a light to moderate pace for 30-60 minutes per exercise session, Group Three is expected to do 3-5 all-out, fast-as-as-you-can-run 100 yard sprints with 3 minutes of rest between efforts.

If we assume three mandatory exercise sessions per week, Group Two is putting in (optimally) a total of three hours of training per week.

Group Three, once we minus out the rest time between HIT intervals, is training 4.5 minutes per week if they only do three sprints per session, or 7.5 minutes per week if they opt for 5 sprint intervals per session.

OK, time-management-wise, HIT, or the tough way is way better. You wind up with oodles more time to do what's next on your to-do list even if that next item is just more "Me" time.

But time-management is not our main concern here. We want to know how well these slackers in Group Three did against the disciplined put-the-time-in folks of

To reap the big results in minimum time you've got to redline it.

Group Two in measures of physical improvement.

First, Group One, the do-nothings. How do you think they did? Yeah, no improvement on any fitness scale. No increase in VO2 Max, no gains in strength or stamina at all and zero fat loss.

Group Two, our long-timers? They saw a slight increase in VO2 Max, slight stamina improvement, very little gains in strength and, as for fat loss, not much.

Now for our Group Three slackers. Improvements across the board and these aren't small gains. At the very minimum HIT matches LSD, but more often than not in test after test, trial after trial, match-up after match-up, HIT exceeds the benefits of LSD training by a long shot.

HIT results show up in all modes of physical effort: Running harder and faster is superior to running slower and longer.

Lifting heavier and more explosively with fewer repetitions is vastly superior to lifting lighter weights, slowly, with lots and lots of reps.

Fewer repetitions of a difficult exercise are superior to

more repetitions of an easier exercise.

So, the science says we can accomplish more in less time. That's a win-win no matter how you measure it.

"Accomplishing more in less time sounds too good to be true. What's the bad news in this story?"

None. But we've got to acknowledge what the acronym HIT stands for:

H is for HIGH — Meaning high or serious levels of output.

I is for INTENSITY — To reap the big results in minimum time you've got to redline it. There is no cruising in this type of training. You can't just strap on your iPod and trot around the neighborhood. If you want the quick results in minimum time, you can't cheat the acronym.

You must train at high intensity and keep your sessions regular. In other words, no "I don't feel like it today because …" Can that stuff and do the work. Keep your focus on the good news, it'll be over soon.

"Won't I have to train like a man to get these results?"

If you want to be tough as we define it in this book, no you don't have to train like a man.

That's good news, right? But …

Men, who get tough don't have to train like men either.

"Wha?"

Men and women who want to get tough need to lose the idea of "this is what boys do" and "this is what girls do" and simply do what athletes do.

I fail to see how a pushup or a pull-up or a sit-up or any inert piece of iron is imbued with gender specific qualities that render it off limits to the opposite sex.

If we recall the wisdom of treating men and women like their weight classes and not their genders and simply scale our workload to the corresponding weight classes and fitness levels, we are finally approaching the topic with some common sense.

"I'll admit that fast results in minimum time sounds good, but I just don't think I'm up to working that hard."

I know that's not a question, but let's treat it as one. The good news about HIT training is that it is all scalable.

What I mean by scalable is that HIT requires you to redline your efforts at all times, but redlines are completely subjective.

My 100 yard sprint may be a walk-in-the-park pace to you. No worries, I still reap the excellent results.

You may be able to power clean only 75 pounds,

> **Men and women who want to get tough need to lose the idea of "this is what boys do" and "this is what girls do" and simply do what athletes do.**

which may seem ridiculously low to another, but that's OK, you'll still have the science on your side.

Whatever the task, as long as you give it all you've got with your current level of intensity, the method will work for you.

Another good thing about HIT redlines is that they are movable. As you adopt the HIT method, your redline will tick upward as your fitness improves.

It is by always pushing that we realize setting the bar higher and higher is what gives us our results and our rewards.

"You make a good case for HIT, but I see some mighty lean ladies wearing yoga pants, so doesn't that mean that low-intensity work is just as effective?"

Not by a long shot.

Look at it this way. Yoga (and even yoga pants) are often self-selecting. I mean those with a figure that is

> ... if exercise of one part of the body led to significant "slimming" or increased muscle size in that area alone, we'd see some pretty bizarre looking athletes out there.

conducive to wearing yoga pants in public will purchase and wear yoga pants in public. (Please, recall one of the top manufacturers of this garment refuses to make or sell sizes above a certain number to continue to perpetuate this lean brand mystique).

Let's look at self-selection in other physical endeavors. Basketball. Lots of tall folks, aren't there? Now, did basketball make them tall or did the nature of the game select for tallness?

Gymnastics. The nature of that sport selects for small-framed light human beings (even in the male divisions). When was the last time you saw an Olympic gymnast who was of NBA basketball height? Again, did gymnastics make these people small or did diminutive people gravitate toward the sport?

With that in mind, I toss out the idea that a product that is made only for slimmer, leaner folks self-selects our thoughts to assume that the yoga did the job of what's filling the pants rather than the product and activity marketing selecting for the pants-fillers.

But if you want to try an experiment via science as we have been doing, hit yoga for 90 days and then compare it with 90 days of HIT training and see which one gets you in those pants sooner.

You already know which one that me and the empirical evidence says will do the job.

"Yeah, I hear you about intensity and time-saving, and all the sciency sort of thing, but what I'm really interested in is toning up my butt, and losing a little off my tummy. Why would I need to do all of these other tough exercises that don't even touch these areas?"

Ah, the old "spot-reducing" business. The thinking goes along these lines: "I'd like to lose some fat off of my belly so I'll do lots and lots of sit-ups, crunches, planks, (insert core exercise of choice) and that will do the trick."

Sounds good in theory, but the reality is the human body does not operate in that manner.

The body is a complex interconnected whole. Just as you can't eat a BLT hold-the-mayo and use the force of your mind to will which part of the body those sandwich calories go to, you can't exercise one small part of your body and expect it to have a slimming effect on that intended target. Oh, if it were that easy.

Look at it this way, if exercise of one part of the body

led to significant "slimming" or increased muscle size in that area alone, we'd see some pretty bizarre looking athletes out there.

Think of tennis players. These are athletes who are either right or left handed and swing that racket with maximum force day in and day out with only one arm.

The last time you watched the US Open did you see the Williams sisters striding the court with one giant arm and one withered arm?

Nope, that's because the human body reads effort and codes that effort by its own standards. Professional tennis players have equally developed arm and shoulder musculature not because of equal effort put in on both sides despite a great deal of effort inequality.

Shelve notions of spot reducing and target slimming and go with what science says works — HIT training.

The good news about HIT training is that it provides results that you desire without specific targeting. Yes, HIT is tougher than an extended crunch session, but it will do the job quickly and efficiently.

By the way, beyond developing and maintaining tennis skills, what method do you think these tennis pros (and all other pro athletes for that matter) are doing to build their conditioning and physiques? Yep, HIT training, the very thing we'll be doing with this manual.

That's the end of our Q & A. Now for some of those

> The good news about HIT training is that it provides just the results that you desire without specific targeting.

sources if you want to look into the science further.

Which Comes First, Cardio or Weights? Fitness Myths, Training Truths and Other Surprising Studies from the Science of Exercise Alex Hutchinson.

The First 20 Minutes: Surprising Science Reveals How We Can Exercise Better, Train Smarter, Live Longer Gretchen Reynolds.

Wrong: Why experts keep failing — and how to know when not to trust them David H. Freedman.
While not a book specifically about training (really, it has nothing to do with it) it is my favorite of the bunch because it opens our eyes to how much of what we consume and presume to be pertinent info may be based in zip. Most useful.

> There are more diets and magic answers shouting for space than actual athletes to adhere to them.

2.1 The Skinny On What Makes Folks Skinny

"He did not sacrifice his health to idle rumours."
— Cicero De Officiis

We are almost to the let's get going portion of the book, but we've got to address the elephant in the room — how to eat so you don't approach the size of an elephant. This is a touchy area. There are more diets and magic answers shouting for space than actual athletes to adhere to them.

Folks grab hold of a diet with the fervency of a new religion and hang on to it forgetting the last diet they just as fervently held on to two years ago. The one they read about in some magazine that Jennifer Aniston was doing to get beach-ready ... or was it Courtney Cox?

Rough waters ahead for true believers, but I've got an ace in the hole — I get to get out of possibly dissing your pet eating superstition. My husband addressed this subject in a prior book. I'll let him take the heat for what we do or don't do in the kitchen.

2 2 What to Eat

by Mark Hatmaker from *Mud, Guts & Glory*

Super secret high performance nutrition

Chances are since you are reading a book about physical activity, you already engage in some form of physical conditioning to bolster your sport performance. I would also wager that if you are serious about your training to any degree, you have some pretty specific ideas regarding nutritional intake. You might be a Paleo-enthusiast in one of its many forms or possibly you're still hanging on to the Zone or the South Beach Diet. Maybe you're an old schooler and an Atkins' proselytizer. Perhaps you're a low fat proponent. Or is it high fat? Do you go for the carbs and carbo load or adhere to the Okinawa protocol? The Mediterranean diet? Are you a strict vegetarian or an all-meat, grass-fed, I-shot-it-myself carnivore.

If I missed your particular take on fuel, I would still place a bet that it is a subdivision or variant of the above panoply. After all, there are only so many ways to juggle the proportions of the three primary constituents of nutrition — protein, carbohydrates and fat.

I will also wager that you've got some pretty good reasons for why you eat what you do and why those who don't follow the same path are a bit misled and not living up to their full potential. Forgive me if this estimation sounds a bit dismissive, but, let's face it, many of us place a lot of faith in the foods we eat imbuing them with qualities that seem to fall short of magical for the "good" foods and bad juju for the "no-no" foods. I've been there myself. I've been a vegan (in a variety of forms), a food-combiner, a low-carber, an all-meat guy, a this-er, a that-er, a fellow searcher who knew that if I got the dinner plate alchemy just right, I would be that much faster, this much stronger, have this much more endurance.

I could find proof for the success of each faith-based path of nutritional wisdom I aligned myself with at the time. I could point to good "science" that supported the belief du jour (while conveniently ignoring the null hypotheses). I could lean hard on my own anecdotal evidence of personal feelings about each awesome diet. I could point to performance numbers showing improvements in tasks and somehow downplay or ignore the idea that these improvements in performance had less to do with the actual training and more to do with what I chewed or what supplement I popped.

I will wager that my experience is shared by many of you. You've either been on this search for the "right thing" treadmill yourself or have personal experience with fellow athletes who pursue a variety of nutritional religions, which we all treat with short memories as soon as we become converted to the next true thing.

Like I said, I've been there, done that and have come to a simple, good news conclusion regarding the art of eating: It's the work — not what you eat.

Wanna eat a large cheese pizza? How about chocolate chip pancakes? Bowls of grits? Pasta? Pop-Tarts? Ben & Jerry's Cheesecake Brownie Ice Cream? How about

It's the work — not what you eat.

beer? (Now that got your attention.)

These are just some of the foods that appeared on the menus of 2012 Olympic athletes. These are not off-season, out-of-training foods. These are truly Olympian food choices. Not food splurges or "cheat day" foods. These aren't even isolated "Oh, I had these four slices of French toast so I'd better not have anything else" foods. These are just some of the so-called "junk foods" that the best of the best consume in a 6,000 calorie day, look-at-me-I'm still-ripped-to-shreds-like-a-superhero regimen. Candy bars, cookies, pizza and beer. How's that for supplementation?

Sure, there are some Olympic athletes who consume their calories in ways that more resemble those listed in the opening paragraph — carefully measured "correct" foods. But what we've got to keep in mind is that those who eat "junk," those who eat "right," those who eat carbs, those who eat meat, those who eat according to whatever belief, all performed at levels beyond the expectations of the common person either because of or in spite of their food choices.

So what if it isn't necessarily what we chow down that's the magic formula? If it's not a one-size-fits-all elite nutrition program that is the secret to Olympic caliber performance or aesthetics, what exactly is it that all of these top-performing athletes have in common? Well, the answer is hard qualitative work in

> **It is possible to eat lots of so-called bad foods and still be a lean, mean, hard-charging athlete, but you gotta work H-A-R-D to get away with it.**

high quantities. And it is this fact of hard, hard grueling work that causes a lot of the magic food ideas to begin to take root.

Composing a shopping list and resisting a few no-no food items while sticking to those foods with good ju-ju is a far, far easier job than pushing the body to extremes. We are economical animals and look for easy/cheap solutions whenever and wherever possible, and there's no seemingly cheaper or easier answer to elite fitness than magic food. If I can get the magic potion just right, the menu tweaked just so, then I too can be golden.

Unfortunately, the evidence says this just isn't true. You can cast about for evidence to support practically any side of the performance nutrition morass and find reams of bolstering information. On the other hand you can find just as much evidence to tear down much of the positive support you can find for the view you wish to support.

These 6,000 calorie-a-day athletes, whether on so called

junk food or healthy diets, put in enormous amounts of strenuous work. (I quibble with the word "junk" as it pertains to food. Tell a starving citizen of a third world nation that a Twinkie is garbage and a poor health choice, and then after that bit of cruelty, see if you can realign your priorities a bit). This prodigious amount of work supports a calories in/calories out model no matter the source of the calories. Those starving in some regions of the world are stark evidence that if you kill those calories, the weight comes off whether you want it to or not.

Let's face it, we aren't Olympic athletes and our workloads simply will not justify 6,000 calories per day no matter their source. But it seems that whether we use the models of Olympic consumption or our own anecdotal evidence of being on this diet or that diet and our body still doing what it does, as long as the work load is of high quality, we can be a bit less dogmatic about what we eat. We don't have to go candy shop crazy since we are not doing Olympic caliber work, but we do have more latitude about what we consume than many of us believe.

For weight control we've got two ways to go. We can adjust caloric intake up or down or we can adjust workload up or down. The optimum mix is to tweak both avenues simultaneously. For some, this info is going to be great news — it appears to allow hardworking athletes a longer leash in regard to food.

For some, this info may be bad news in two ways. It is possible to eat lots of so-called bad foods and still be a lean, mean, hard-charging athlete, but you gotta work

H-A-R-D to get away with it. You can't shortcut the work. Some will remain happier with the easier job of composing restrictive grocery shopping lists.

The second way the info may be a bit of bad news is that if you are firmly committed to your "scientifically proven high-performance nutrition program" du jour, the cognitive dissonance may make eating whatever you damn well please as long as you are willing to do the work a bit hard to swallow.

I get that skepticism. Those immersed in physical training are (and always have been) confronted with conflicting fuel ideas every which way they turn. How could there not be something to it? I point again to Olympic diets whether deemed good, bad or indifferent, and again to the similarity of excellent results and see that the only commonality is eating enough calories to support your workload and then burn those calories off with ultra-high quality work.

> "I love apple pie. If I see one, I'm going to eat the whole thing."
>
> — Rich Froning, Three-time CrossFit Champion

2.3 Sometimes You Can Have Your Apple Pie and Eat It Too

The preceding should have been mighty encouraging news regarding food. I mean, when you get down to it, who wants to work H-A-R-D and eat like a bird or a medical patient? After all that hard work don't we deserve to treat ourselves right?

I think so.

And here's yet another person who thinks the same thing: Rich Froning.

Who's he?

According to CrossFit, Rich Froning is The Fittest Man in the World having racked up three CrossFit Games World Championships in a row. In an interview with *Outside Magazine* conducted by Gordy Megroz, Mr. Fittest Man in the World has this to say:

Screw Diets!
"A lot of people who do CrossFit eat a strict paleo diet, but I don't subscribe to any specific way of eating. If you burn enough calories, you don't need to."

> **Skip the work and you might need to say hello to a nice glass of water and a stick of celery.**

Sweets Are OK!
"I love apple pie. If I see one, I'm going to eat the whole thing."

What did I tell you? Do the work and you can still enjoy your life. Let's stop being slaves to grocery list taboos and religious adherents of dinner plate wisdom.

If you'd like to hear more of Mr. Froning's common sense have a look here:
http://www.outsideonline.com/fitness/strength-and-power-training/Pro-Tips-CrossFit-Champ-Rich-Froning.html

And in case you're wondering do I eat what I preach? Yep.

For example, my husband and I love obstacle course runs — Spartan Races, Rugged Maniacs, Mudathlon, those sorts of things.

Pre-race breakfast is almost invariably a candy bar: Snickers for me, a Payday for him.

Post-race meal is always a big bag of fast food chowed down in the car on the way home (usually KFC, Taco Bell or any food truck we can find with burritos the size of your thigh.

One more time, if you put the work in you can cut yourself some slack.

Skip the work and you might need to say hello to a nice glass of water and a stick of celery.

Mmm, yum!

3. One is the Loneliest Number

One of the best ways to keep motivated for the work you want to do is to have a training partner or partners.

Me? I'm lucky to always have my husband to work with, plus or minus whatever clients are in for a grueling little MMA visit.

Having a partner to work alongside of, to compete or race against, to cheer on or to good naturedly trash talk (I'm talking to you, Dan "Scrub" Marx) does wonders for your motivation.

If you can find kindred spirits in pursuing this program, I say the more the merrier — just make sure that each member of your crew purchases separate copies of this book so they can fully absorb the material. For best results, two copies apiece is advised.

But don't let lack of a training partner, or partner(s) unable to make this or that session dependent on whether or not you do the work.

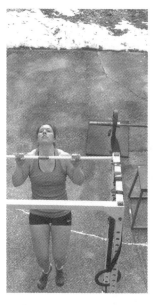

Yes, more than one can make it a bit more fun, but one (and that one being you) is more than enough to get the job done.

Don't let anybody else's motivation, or lack thereof, be your excuse for not being motivated.

Whether anyone is sweating along with you or not, you will always reap the rewards of what you do — nobody's work but yours will make you better.

And if you want virtual/on-line support as you work through this manual, feel free to visit my site and let me and others like you know how you are doing. With or without training partner(s), you'll find nothing but team camaraderie and solidarity here.

Cosmonot.us
Facebook.com/kylie.cosmonot

4.1 Get with the Program

How to read the workouts

We're just a few pages away from actually breaking a sweat, just a few more logistics to get out of the way to make sure you get the most out of the program.

In the Workout Menu section you will find three separate numbers, or set of numbers following each workout as in the example below:

Pull-ups 10/8/6
Push-ups 10/8/6
Xs 10

The first number following the exercise is the number of repetitions prescribed for the female athlete who has already been training with intensity for at least six months.

The second number is for the female athlete who already does some fitness activities, but is new to intensity training.

The third number is for all of our sisters who are brand spanking new to training, or it's been a long time since you've done such a thing.

So, advanced ladies do 10 reps each of pull-ups and push-ups, our intermediate ladies will be doing 8 reps of each and our rookie friends 6 reps each.

"Xs 10" means times 10 or 10 sets. That is, repeat your rep number for pull-ups and push-ups 10 times.

Anytime you encounter weight exercises the numbers inside the parentheses are the prescribed weights — again in the toughest to rookie order.

Example:
Back squat (135/115/95) 10/8/6
Xs 3

So 3 sets of 10 reps at 135 pounds for advanced, 8 reps at 115 pounds for intermediate and 6 reps at 95 pounds for beginner.

"Countdown" following a workout means your first rep is the stated number, the second is the stated number less one, the third the stated number less two and so on until you get to 1.

Example:
Pull-ups 10/8/6
Squats 10/8/6
Countdown both exercises

The advanced women will do 10 reps of each in their first set, 9 reps of each in their 2nd set, 8 reps in set three and so on until they do their ones.

"Death by ..." (as in "Death by power clean") means that you will set a timer and do 1 repetition of the given exercise in minute one. At minute 2 do 2 reps. At minute 3 do 3 reps and so on until you can't fit the designated repetitions inside the minute (death comes faster than you think).

You will encounter the word "fatigue" as in

Pull-up fatigue 100/75/50

You know what the rep numbers mean, but the word "fatigue" imposes a penalty.

Example:
Pull-up fatigue 100/75/50
Penalty: squats 10/8/6

Our toughest sisters will be required to do 100 pull-ups total, but anytime they come off the bar they will have to perform the penalty exercise and then get right back on the bar with no rest. Even if that next rep is 1 measly rep and right back to the penalty.

Sounds like it sucks doesn't it? It does.

The phrase "Rounds in..." as in

Burpees 10/8/6
Kettlebell swing (55/40/25) 10/8/6
Rounds in 20m

... means you will do the prescribed repetitions and weights getting as many sets/rounds as you can inside the time limit. Here 20m is to be read as 20 minutes.

You will also encounter the initials RM usually preceded by a number as in:

Back squat 5/2s to find your 2RM

RM means Repetition Maximum. This means that all levels have 5 sets of 2 to try to build towards what is your maximum weight that day of 2 repetitions.

Ideally, you will do a moderate start and build toward heavier poundage as you progress through your sets. An example for a rookie might look like:

Set 1: 95 pounds
Set 2: 115 pounds
Set 3: 135 pounds
Set 4: 150 pounds
Set 5: Attempted 160, but only made 1 rep.

4.2 Take It Down a Notch, Never Up

The key to this program is scalability. That is, no matter your fitness level you will be able to jump aboard the wagon going to Texas.

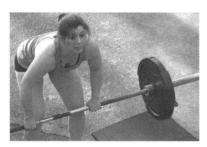

If an exercise is initially too difficult for you, we provide training step options to fill in the gaps until we get to the real thing.

If the rep numbers seem too high in the beginning, it's your call if you want to alter them — think about what you want out of the program before you do, though. Make sure you are scaling down for necessity, not laziness.

If the weight prescription is a tad too high for you, knock it down a bit. No problem.

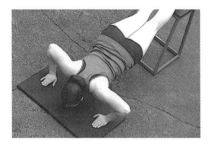

Scalability is always negotiable downward, but ... never scale it up. What I mean is if a pre-scribed weight seems too low, rather than up that weight, your job is to strive to work through that day's challenge faster. Save your heavy weight yearnings for RM days.

Often athletes (male and female) enjoy their newfound strength and want to bump weights higher. But this may work at cross purposes since, yes, there will be intensity at the higher weight, but the recovery required may slow you down in whatever else is in that day's challenge. You may wind up dampening your overall intensity effect without meaning to.

4.3 No to the Same-Old, Same-Old
This program has constant variation with very little repeating sequences as its backbone. Seldom do exact workout challenges repeat themselves. Individual exer-cises will rear their difficult heads time and again in various combinations, but cookie cutter workout tem-plates are few and far between.

The reason for this is found in the phrase "Variety is the spice of life." To work as hard as we are advocating here can get mighty tough when you are dragging your butt out the door for your 100th day of doing the same thing. Tweaking daily workout challenges keeps an intellectual freshness going that is a bit easier to wrap our motivation around.

If you worry that you won't "get good" at anything by varying your challenges constantly and not focusing on a few handfuls of movement, think of educating your body just the way you educate your mind.
To really master an academic subject you don't read the same book again and again and again. You read first this book on the chosen subject, then that book, and then another and yet another. When you master that subject there will be repeating elements in each book as your knowledge progresses, but there is no need to buckle down and read the same book again and again.

For example, who's more well-read: the person who has read Moby Dick 300 times or the person who read Moby Dick and then progressed through 299 other volumes?
It's the same in the physical world. The more physical challenges you are able to adapt to and overcome, the more fit you will be in a broad spectrum as opposed to being good in one tiny area.

Why do any of the challenges repeat at all?

Good question. Read on.

4.4 How Are You Doing?

When you begin your trip to Texas, you're going to start feeling improvements almost immediately. Well,

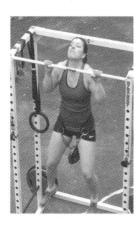

once you get past an initial week to 10 days of "My Lord, am I sore!"

About 30 days out from your start you won't just feel the changes, you'll start seeing them, too.

But sometimes it's nice to have some quantifiable proof of how you're doing. You will have one of three ways to record your progress.

1. Beat the Clock
In any workout you are not striving for an RM, you will set a timer and strive to complete that day's challenge as quickly as possible (with good exercise form of course). Record that time and if/when that specific workout challenge rears its head, compare your new time to your old time. You will always be striving to match or beat that time.

2. Rounds in …
This is another variation of the Beat the Clock score-keeping method. Anytime your workout says Complete Such and Such Rounds in Such and Such Minutes, record your completed rounds. If/when that challenge repeats, strive to match or beat your prior performance.

3. Repetition Maximum

On these days no clock is required. It's just you and the weight and seeing how much you can lift. When these days repeat, you are striving to match or beat.

These three methods are ideal ways to benchmark progress and to add a bit of competition to what you are doing, even though that competition is only against yourself.

Besides, always having a clock to work against makes it into a game — a sort of cognitive destination rather than just another day of grinding gym routine. And destinations are almost always a good thing. Going somewhere is always way more fun and productive than going nowhere.

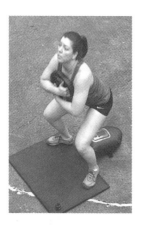

5. Gearing Up to Get Going

Equipment you will need

There are three ways to go when it comes to workout gear:

1. Join a gym and let them cover the gear expenses with your membership fees. Be advised most gyms don't necessarily stock the most useful gear. If they do, they won't take kindly to the hard-use we advocate you putting it through. Believe me, my husband and I while on vacation away from our home gym have been told "Please don't do that" on more than one occasion.

2. Go out of pocket and set up your own home gym.
This is often the ideal way as you are beholding to no
one and can train when your schedule permits. It's
mighty hard to beat the convenience of having your
gym right under your nose. Having a home gym kills
the "I don't have the time" excuse when it's just a few
short steps to the garage.

3. Share gear expenses with training partners. If you
have committed partners, this is a mighty nice way to
defray the costs. But, of course, they need to be as hard
charging as you intend to be.

Of the three ways to get your hands on gear #2 is, as I
already said, ideal, but I recognize that not all of us
have the money or the desire to Donald Trump on our
home gym from the word go. With that in mind, we
offer three approaches for the inspired aspiring tough
girl. You will find suggested gear retailers in the
Resources section.

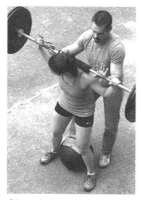

Olympic bar with plates and plates. Plates are held by spring collars.

Bare minimum

For the just getting started, economical approach. You don't have to purchase these all at once. Gradual procurement is fine.

1. This book. Look, you're already on your way!

2. A workout timer or watch with stopwatch function that will allow you to time your workouts. Ideally your timer of choice will also have a countdown function and audible prompts that will allow you to use it on "Rounds in ..." days.

3. A notebook or document file that will allow you to record your daily workout scores for future reference and comparison.

4. Workout clothing of your choice that fits your climate. I have found that fitted garments with stretch do the job. Too loose and you can jump out of them (no kidding, I've done that). Too tight and movement is restricted.

5. Workout footwear. Minimal soles are ideal. Higher soles can lead to rolled ankles on any chal-

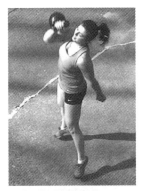

Lifting a kettlebell

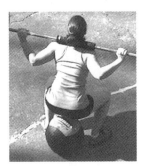

Medicine ball as butt-bumper

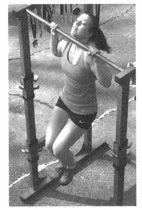

Pull-up bar on a squat cage

lenge that emphasizes lateral movement. Minimal soles also allow you to lift weight with better form. High cushy soles have a tendency to compress when you lift and can possibly lead to ankle or knee instability.

6. An Olympic weight bar with spring collars. The latter hold the weight on and are much faster to use than lock-down collars. A fitted neck pad that can be taken on and off the bar is not essential, but mighty nice to have all the same.

7. A set of Olympic plates. Initially, pairs of 2.5, 5, 10, 25 and 45 pounds should do it.

8. A single kettlebell for your fitness level — 45, 35 and 25 pounds for each respective fitness level.

9. A butt-bumper. This is a cushioned surface to let you know you've dropped low enough on a few exercises. We use a padded medicine ball, but any forgiving surface that is at least 14-15 inches high should do the trick.

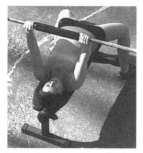

Pressing on a bench

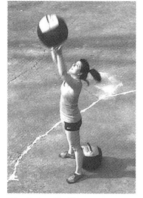

Medicine balls

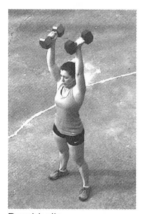

Dumbbells

10. It's a good idea to have floor pads to protect your workout deck from dropped weights.

A step up
All of the above plus:

1. A click counter to keep up with repetitions. I use an Adidas pitch counter that I picked up from Dick's Sporting Goods for $10. Look in the baseball gear section.

2. Another pair of 45 pound Olympic plates.

3. Another kettlebell 10 pounds more than your fitness level be it 55, 45 or 35 pounds.

4. A pull-up bar. If it has a bar dip attachment, even better.

5. A bench for bench press days (these aren't often so don't make this your first purchase).

6. A 20-pound medicine ball.

7. A few pairs of dumbbells to match your fitness level — pairs of 40, 30 and 20 pounds.

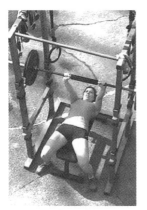

Squat cage or tower

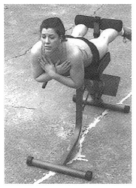

Roman chair

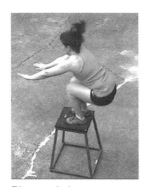

Plyometric box

Whole hog

Everything you'll need to be the best you can be.

All of the preceding plus:

1. Make your Olympic plates bumper plates which are made of solid rubber and are more forgiving when you drop them.

2. A squat cage/rack that will allow you to lift heavy for your class with safety. Make sure it comes with a pull-up bar and dip station. You'll also be able to hang gymnastic rings from this bar for ring dips.

3. A Roman chair and back extension bench.

4. A pair of rings if your goal is to hit ring dips one day.

5. A plyometric box for your fitness level — 24, 20 and 18 inches high, respectively.

6. A dip belt which allows you to attach weight plates to your body for weighted pull-ups and dips.

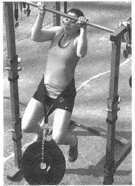

Dip belt with plate

7. A low 12-inch hurdle. Keep in mind you can improvise this item. A 24-inch hurdle might also be nice to have on hand.

8. A 15-foot climbing rope. If you've got no tree, throw it over your pull-up bar.

9. A rolling measure or some other device for calculating sprint distances.

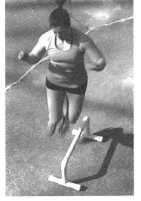

12-inch hurdle

10. A white board (dry erase board) is useful for days with long sequences so you can get a good and easy view of what madness is next in the sequence.

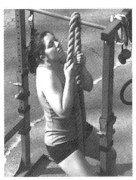

Climbing rope

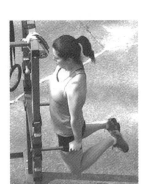

Dip bars on squat cage

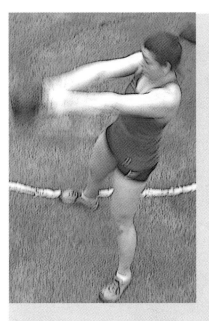

6. She's Tough Exercise Vocabulary

In the following pages you will find each of the individual exercises we use in the program listed alphabetically for easy reference. Even if you think you know what we mean by a given exercise, do me a favor and have a look at it anyway to see if there is a particular standard or point of form we'd like you to use to keep that intensity burning bright.

You will also find a few "But I Can't Do That!" sections where we provide building block exercises (not substitutions) to get you from "No, I can't" to "Yes, I can!"

You can find video demonstrations of many of these on our YouTube channel:

http://www.youtube.com/kyliehatmaker

Back extensions

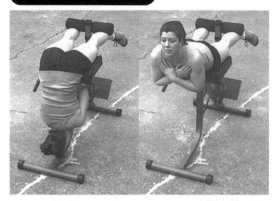

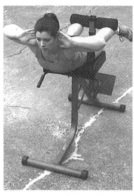 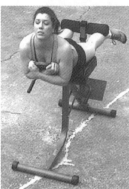

● Place yourself on the back extension bench facing downward.

● Your Achilles tendons will be locked under the foot catch and your hips will rest on the stand.

● Fold your arms across your chest and bend at the waist until you are at a 90 degree bend, flex your glutes and hamstrings to bring yourself back parallel with the floor.

● More advanced versions of this call for
1. Hands behind the head
2. Holding a weight plate to your chest.

Back pedal

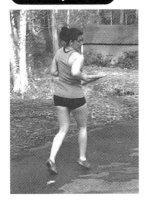 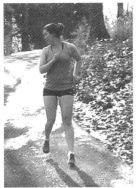

This is simply running backward. We use the back pedal to activate different musculature than standard running does. Hit hills with a back pedal and the fronts of your thighs and hips will light up with a white hot burn.

Back squat

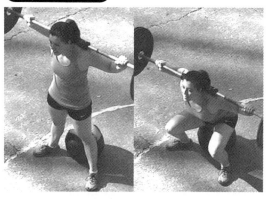

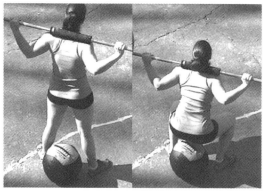

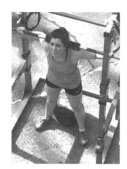
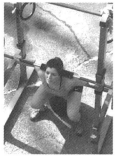

For heavy weight use a rack for stability. The images above and throughout the text are sans rack to better show technique.

- One of the Queen Maker exercises. Developing a good squat will lead to large strides in your fitness because it makes so many demands on your musculature.
- Place an Olympic bar (O-bar from here on out) on the rack approximately 2 inches below your shoulder height.
- Place your butt-bumper on the ground.
- Step beneath the bar to rack the bar across the back of your shoulders.
- To rack the bar don't simply lay the bar across passive shoulders, instead, think of hunching your shoulders backward and upward as if you were going to pinch a quarter between your shoulder blades. Rack the bar across this "pinched" position.
- Keeping the pinched position throughout, grip the bar with both hands pulling it into your pinched shoulders.
- Take a stance just slightly wider than shoulder width apart.
- Keep your head up throughout and lower back flat, descend to the butt-bumper.
- To come back to standing, don't think of just standing up, but pushing your feet toward the outside as if you were standing on a large sheet of tearable paper and you wanted to rip it apart (although you are thinking of spreading your feet, they won't actually move)
- A common squat error is to lean or bend forward at the waist — particularly at the bottom of the exercise. This places undue stress on the back and takes you out of balance. If you picture the exercise from a profile you are striving to keep the bar centered as close to over your heels as you can throughout the movement.

Side bar
"What the heck is a butt-bumper?"
A butt-bumper is any cushioned prop approximately 14-15 inches high that you can place on the ground beneath your hips. The purpose of the bumper is not to have a seat on it and rest, but to let you know when you have dropped low enough to build intensity and strength in your squat. Hedge the bet and stop short you are doing only a fraction of the work. You're not gonna get to Texas by doing that. I use a large 20# medicine ball as a butt-bumper.

Bench press

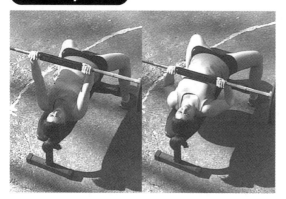

● Lie back on the bench and place your eyes just beneath the bar. If the bar is too far rearward or forward, you'll make it tough to get the bar into position.

● Hit the shoulder pinch position that you did in the back squat — this helps keep the back tight. Even though you are using your chest, we call on more physiological resources by tightening head to toe.

● Place your feet flat on the floor and think of dragging your heels back toward your shoulders. Again, they won't actually move, we are just recruiting more muscle.

● Place your hands on the O-bar approximately shoulder width apart and lock your elbows.

● You will then lower the bar to your chest (around the nipple line) with your elbows traveling outward from the body — not necessarily at an extreme angle just not tucked in close.

● Keeping your shoulders pinched and your heels dragging, fire the bar back to elbows locked position.

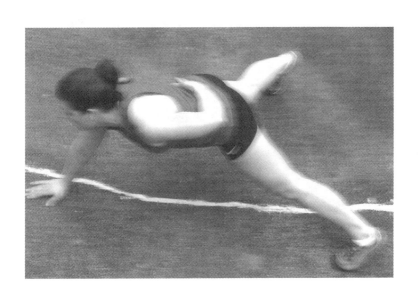

Box jump

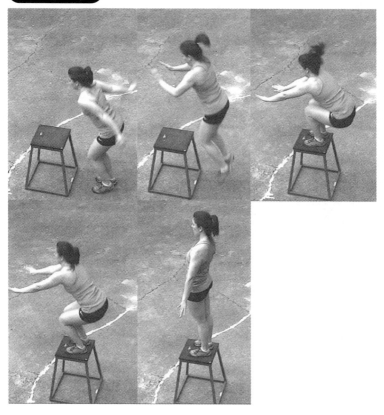

- Place yourself in front of the box with your feet shoulder width apart.
- Descend to a quarter squat and use an aggressive arm swing as you jump bringing your knees to your chest to land on top of the box.
- Once on the box, come to a complete stand before jumping backward off the box landing in a quarter squat to absorb the impact.

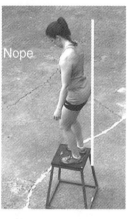

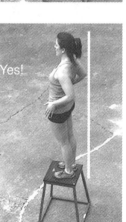

Side Bar

"You keep referring to a full-stand, are you implying that I may be standing wrong?"

Maybe.

There's a tendency in repetitive squat/jumping exercises to mistake knees locked but bent forward at the waist as a full stand. What we want for good form is rising to knees locked, hips pushed forward and shoulders back. When we're working with a partner and we see standing form deteriorate, we give a call of "Hips-thru!" to remind ourselves to get the technique right.

Burpees

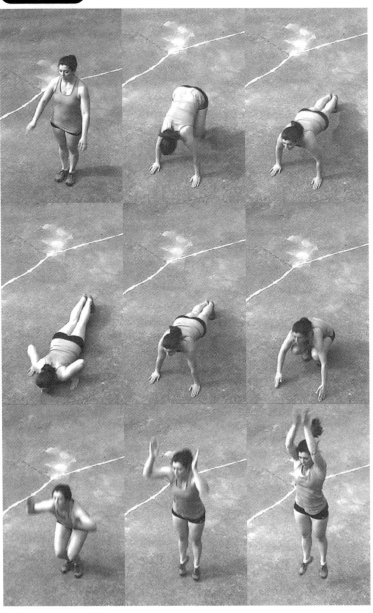

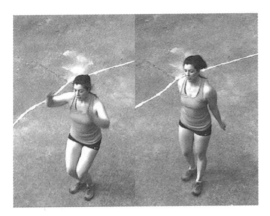

● This is a full body burner. If it's raining out and you don't feel like running, this will get the heart and lungs pumping.

● From a standing position, jump/sprawl your feet backward until you land in a push-up position.

● Drop and hit one push-up — head up, chest and upper thighs touching the ground.

● At the top of the push-up, jump your feet back beneath you.

● As you stand, jump approximately 6-8 inches off of the ground and clap your hands overhead.

● That's one rep.

Can't do a full push-up? See the push-up section for help in building that bad boy.

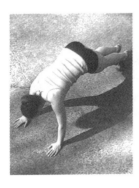
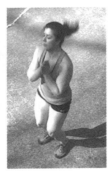

Common bad from left to right. Keep the butt down during push-ups. Jump up, extend and clap overhead with intent when you finish each rep.

Clean & jerk

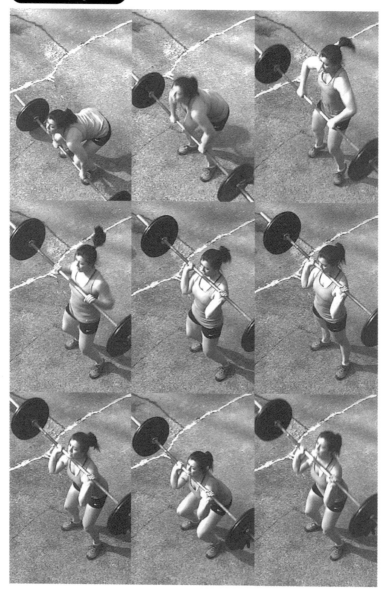

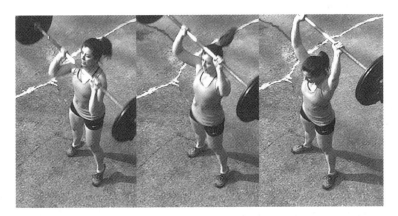

This is a two part exercise. See the explanation of the power clean for details on how to execute part one.

● To execute the jerk, we'll assume you already have the bar in clean position (held at collarbone level).

● The following all happens simultaneously: Drop to a quarter squat underneath the bar and drive the bar upward (dropping while driving allows you to get underneath weight you can't strictly press under normal conditions).

● Once the bar is locked out overhead, walk your feet back underneath you to shoulder width.

● Drop the bar to the ground — that's one rep.

Side bar
"What is a Proof of Lift (POL)?"

Proof of lift is nothing more than a brief pause at the top of the lift to prove/show that you are in control of the weight. The POL pause need last no more than a second and should be used in all weighted exercises.

Dead lift

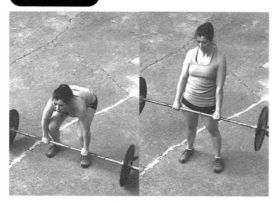

● Another Queen maker.

● With the O-bar on the ground, stand with your feet at shoulder width and your toes underneath the bar. When you look down you should see the bar "cutting your foot in half."

● Grip the bar at shoulder width with either a standard grip or a flipped grip.

● You will be in a quarter squat position with your head up and your back flat. Push through your heels (not your toes) and pull/lift the bar until you hit a full stand — back straight, shoulders back, and hips pushed forward.

● If you think pushing through your heels and "jumping backward" rather than lifting, you're on the right track.

Dips

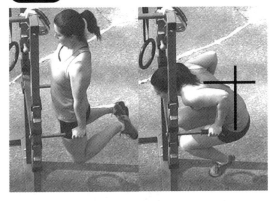

● You will use a fixed dip station for this exercise — the more difficult version uses gymnastic rings.
● Grip the bars with your head up, elbows locked and shoulders in pinched position.
● Lower yourself until your elbows are at 90 degrees — striving to keep your shoulders pinched throughout.
● Squeeze your elbows toward your body as you drive your body back to the top of the locked position.

Side bar
"But I can't do dips!"

No worries, you are not alone. One of the little differences between the male and female of the species is muscle mass. Pound for pound we simply lack the same amount of muscle in the upper body as a similarly sized male. We have to work just a wee bit harder at some exercises, dips being one of them.

Another little biological difference is a bit of skeletal engineering. Men's arms when locked straight form an almost perfect line, whereas when we ladies lock our arms you will notice a slight outward angle from the elbow to the wrist. This outward swoop was evolution's answer to our wider hips. If we had the straight arms of men we would be bumping into ourselves with each swing of the arms while walking. *Continued next page.*

Continued from previous page.

This angled feature of the human body does make it slightly less efficient for pushing in the locked arm position for a dip, but it can be done.

I've provided some "This will get you there ..." exercises below.

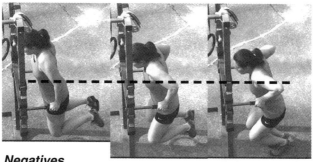

Negatives

● In this training version of the dip, you will start at full locked out position and lower yourself as slowly and painfully as possible to the 90 degree position.

● At the bottom of the 90 degrees make no effort to return to the top, simply put your feet down and start at the top again.

● The key is to go s-l-o-w-l-y.

● Count each negative as that day's rep.

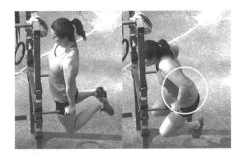

Partials
● Exactly what it sounds like — get on the bar and descend to the point where you feel that you may lose control, then return to position.
● Count each partial as one full repetition with the goal that each dip session will see you being able to descend a bit lower than the last.

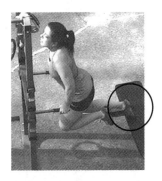

Foot assist
● In this version, you will hit the full range of motion, but you will have an assist in the form of a bench or plyo box.
● Hit the locked out position and place one foot (just one!) toes down on your assist device.
● Descend with control using only the amount of assist from the foot prop. Return to locked out position.

Elbow hitch pull-ups

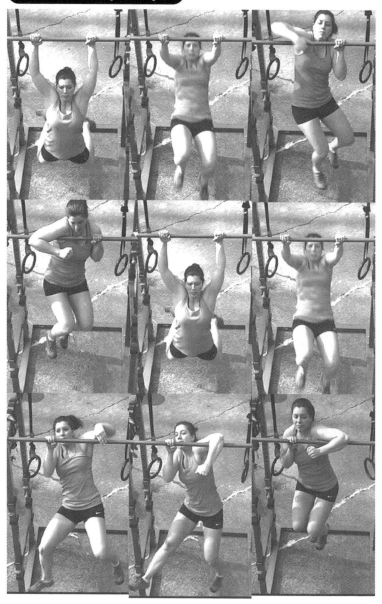

This is a pull-up variant we use sometimes that is an ideal functional exercise for all of you out there who enjoy obstacle course races and need some powerful help to get over high walls.

● For pull-up training steps see *"But I can't do pull-ups!"* in the pull-up section.
● From a dead hang on the bar, hit a hard fast surge and rise until you can take your right arm off of the bar and throw it over the bar bringing yourself to a temporary stop at the top of the motion.
● Regrip, drop down and surge back up for a repetition on the opposite side.

Front squat

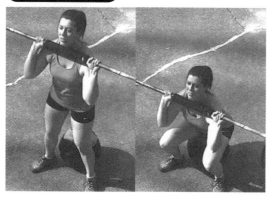 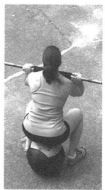

● Place your O-bar on the rack at approximate shoulder level.

● Place your butt-bumper beneath your hips.

● Step under the bar and place it in clean position — bar at your collarbone level.

● You will use the same mechanics to hit the front squat as you do the back squat. The difference being that with the weight loaded to the front of your body you will need to be all the more scrupulous about keeping your back straight and your posture upright. There is a big tendency to lean forward at the bottom which will cause you to pitch the weight forward.

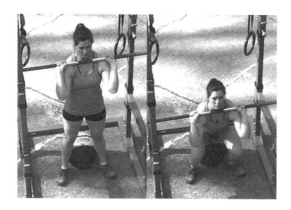

Ground to overhead

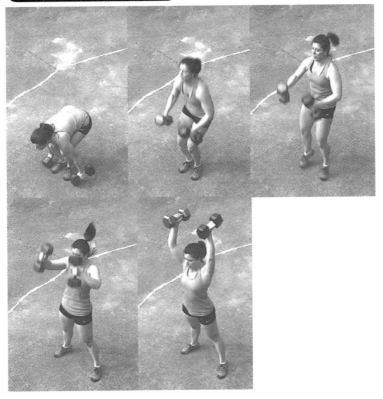

Anytime you encounter the workout challenge "Ground to Overhead" it is understood that you are to move whatever the object is (dumbbells, O-bar, kettlebell, et cetera) from the ground to overhead.

● You can use whatever method you desire — swing, clean and jerk, snatch, whatever as long as it is just you struggling with the weight. Touch the weight at the bottom and hit POL at the top.

Hang clean

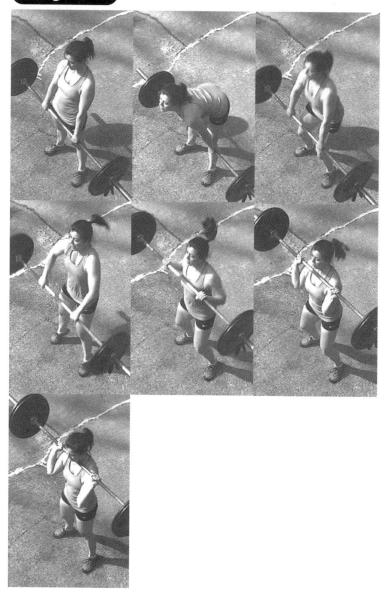

- This is a great exercise for building explosive power.
- Grip an O-bar and hold it at arm's length in front of your hips.
- Simultaneously hit a quarter squat and a quick backward shrug with your shoulder blades to jump under the bar into clean position.

Side bar
"The power ends when the elbow bends."

In approaching any weight exercise, it is ideal if you think of it not as weight lifting but as weight throwing. The difference may sound subtle, but in application it is not. We don't want slow controlled lifts. We are aiming at using good form to throw the weight into the positions we desire — building both strength and power at the same time.

To assist us in being more effective when throwing weights, it is useful to keep the phrase "The power ends when the elbow bends" in mind.

In all of our lifts we want to recruit our legs and hips to do the majority of the job as these are the most powerful parts of the body. To make sure we are utilizing our legs and hips to the utmost and not trying to "muscle" the weight with our upper body, we strive to do 90 percent of our lifts with our legs and hips leaving the elbows straight until the last 10 percent of the motion.

The power surges from the soles of our feet, through our knees, then our hips, through an aggressive shoulder-pinch/shrug and finally (and only then) through a bend in the elbows.

This is a subtle point, but it makes a huge difference.

Hang squat clean

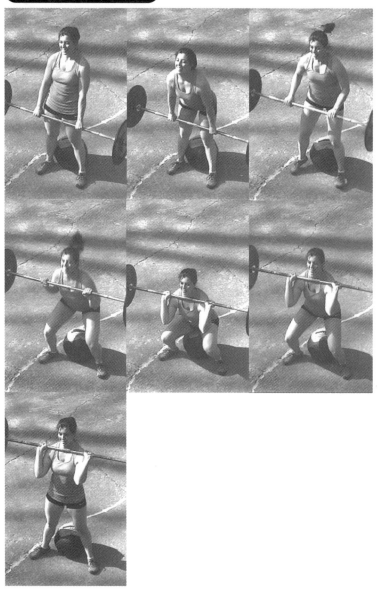

● Think of this as a combination front squat and hang clean.
Hit the hang clean with the
addition of dropping into a
squat onto a butt-bumper and
then rising to a full stand with a
front squat.

● Notice we are jumping
underneath the bar into the full
squat, not hitting the hang
clean and then dropping to the
butt-bumper.

Kettlebell clean & jerk

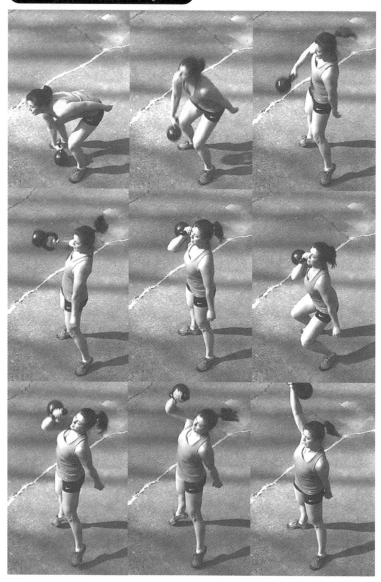

● This is the same mechanics as the O-bar clean and jerk, but using either a single kettlebell or two kettlebells as that day's challenge specifies.

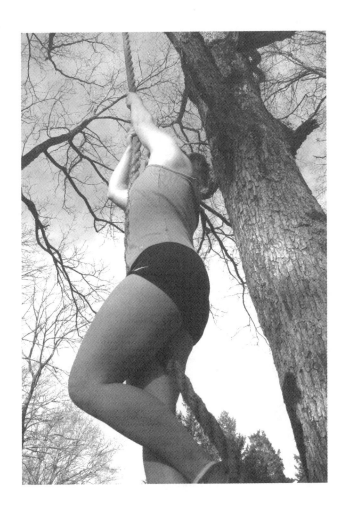

Kettlebell swing

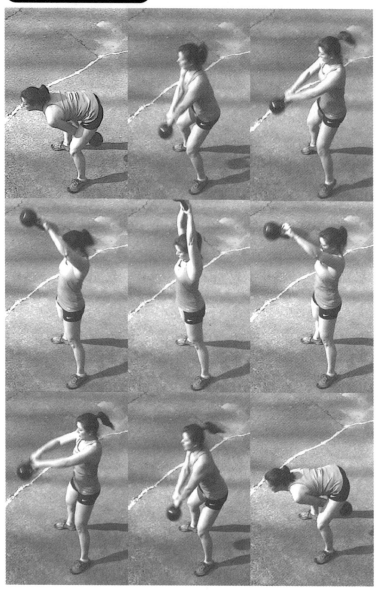

- Straddle the kettlebell (KB from here on out) with your feet a little wider than shoulder's width apart.
- Keeping your back straight and shoulder's pinched, drop and grip the KB handle with both hands.
- You will explode forward with your hips and rise to a full stand as you swing the KB to an overhead position — back straight and hips through, defined as pushed forward.
- As the KB travels back downward, hit that quarter squat and block your forearms with your inner thighs launching you into your next repetition.
- Keep in mind, as with most all of our lifts, we want the legs, hips, and shoulder pinch to precede and augment what we do with our arms and shoulders.
- Note: I find that the brief inertial pause at the top of the motion is a nice spot to take a needed breath.

Knees to elbows

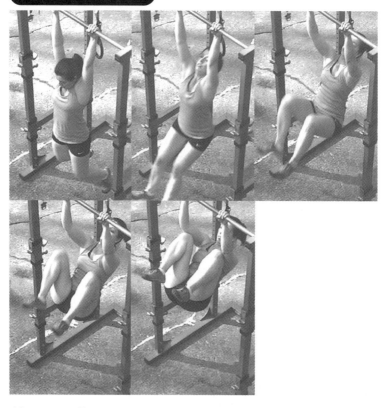

Knees to elbows
● Grip your pull-up bar with your arms at dead-hang position.
● Tuck your legs and rock backward while giving a slight pull
with your arms until each knee touches the respective elbow.

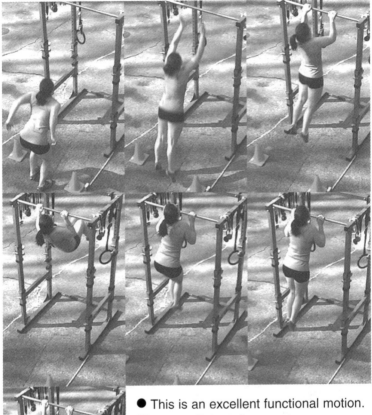

● This is an excellent functional motion. (If you can't do pull-ups yet, see our helping exercises in the pull-up section.)
● Mark a line 3 feet away from your pull-up bar.
● From behind that line take a leap, catch the bar in both hands and strive to pull your chin above the bar from this ballistic entry.
● Drop off the bar, go back behind the line and repeat.

Low hurdle hops

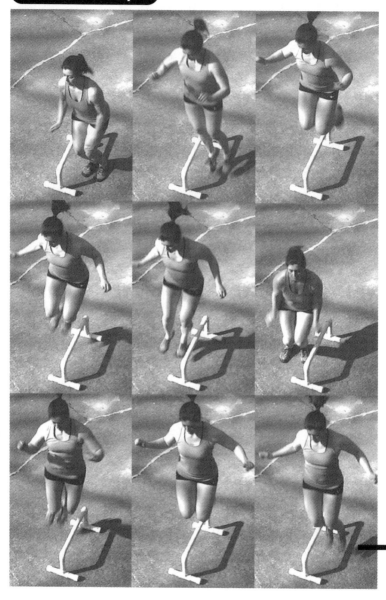

- Place your low-hurdle (any 12 inch barrier will do) on the ground.
- Stand perpendicular to the hurdle.
- Rapidly hop to the other side always using a two-footed hop with the feet close together (not merely stepping over the hurdle).
- We are striving for rapid back and forth hops, crew!

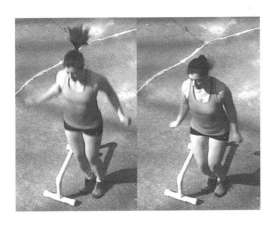

One arm push-ups

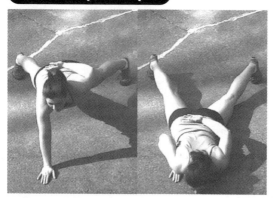

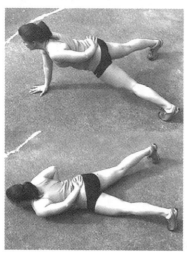

● This is a nice change-up and a big confidence builder once you've finally mastered push-ups.
● I find taking a little wider stance with my feet …
● Tightening my core hard …
● And tucking my elbow tight to my body as I push helps.

Overhead squat

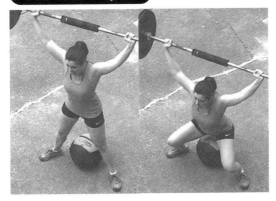

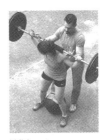

Without a cage you'll need a spotter for sure.

● A tough, tough, tough exercise.

● Place your O-bar on the rack at shoulder level and your butt-bumper on the floor.

● Step under the bar and place it on your pinched shoulders.

● Stand over your butt-bumper with a stance that is approximately two shoulder widths apart.

● Spread your hands on the bar to approximately the same width as your feet.

● Give a short burst from the legs to lock the bar overhead — now, we start the exercise.

● Your job is to keep the bar in overhead lockout position as you drop to your butt-bumper and return to a full stand.

● It will help to recall the mechanics of the back squat— keeping the overhead bar lined up over your hips and heels throughout the motion will cure most of what ails you.

● A profile view reveals that your arms and shoulders must travel a bit rearward to keep the proper alignment. It may look a little weird from the outside, but it does the trick.

● There is a huge tendency to shift the weight forward as you descend. But if you don't defeat this tendency, you will never keep any significant weight overhead. Be scrupulous with your form from the beginning and you'll make huge strides.

Power clean

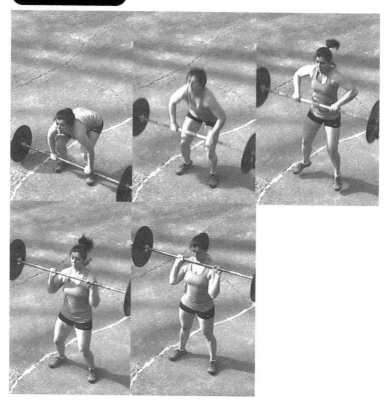

● A foundation exercise.
● With your O-bar on the ground, stand before it with feet at shoulder's width.
● Keeping your back flat and head up, squat and grip the bar at a shoulder's width.
● Keeping "the power ends when the elbow bends" in mind, jump and throw the bar to clean position — held at collarbone level.

Prisoner squats

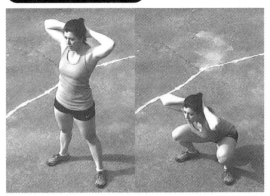

Good form — head up and back straight.

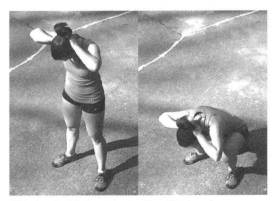

This is what fatigue looks like. Buck up!

● This is a back squat with no weight — but don't go thinking it's easy. We use high reps on this exercise to get that burn going deep.

● Place your your butt-bumper on the ground, straddle it and place your hands behind your head.

● Drop to the bumper and rise — keeping your head up and back straight throughout. There will be a tendency to want to pull the head down with your hands as you get tired. Resist it, ladies!

Pull-ups (strict)

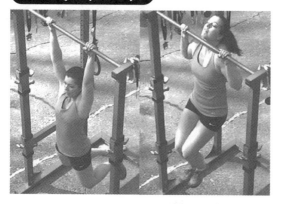

- Grip the bar with a shoulder width grip — arms at full extension — no partially bent elbows to cheat your way up.
- Pull yourself to the bar until your chin is above it.
- Drop to a dead hang and repeat.

Side bar
"But I can't do pull-ups!"

This is a difficult exercise for women for some of the same reasons that dips are difficult. But with the following steps, there is no reason in the world why you can't build to true pull-ups with some Texas-sized diligence.

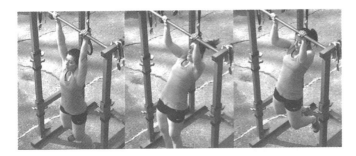

Partials
● Grip the bar and give it what you've got, even if you only move 2-3 inches from the bottom. Count that as a step in the right direction.
● Next pull-up day strive to wriggle up a little further.

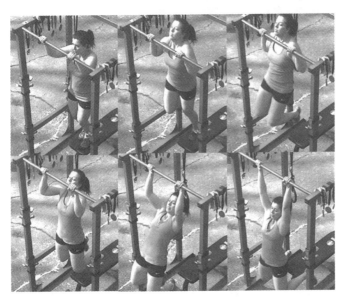

Negatives
● Place a plyo box beneath the bar and start at the top of the motion.
● Once at the top, step off of the box and descend as slowly as possible.
● Once at a full dead hang, use the box to get back to the top and repeat.

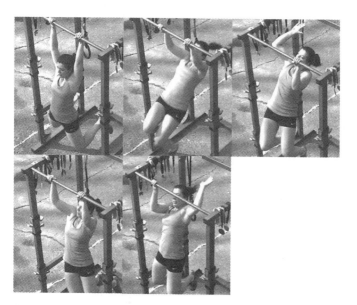

Hot bar

● Often the toughest portion of the pull-up to educate is the surge needed from the very bottom of the exercise. I use the hot bar training step to build the surge required.

● From your full dead hang, surge hard and fast and quickly take one hand off of the bar for a fraction of a second and then quickly re-grip the bar.

● On your next repetition do a quick release with the opposite hand and so on and so forth.

PULL-UPS PART DEAUX

Kipping pull-ups

● Once you have mastered the pull-up, you are more than welcome to use a kipping motion to get to the top of the bar.

● There are many ways to kip, but think of it essentially as any wriggle, leg kick or coordinated hip swing that gets you from dead hang to the top of the bar.

● Anytime you see a workout posted as pull-ups, assume you are allowed to kip unless a strict pull-up is prescribed for that day's challenge.

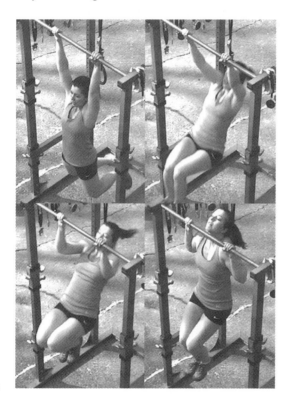

Push press

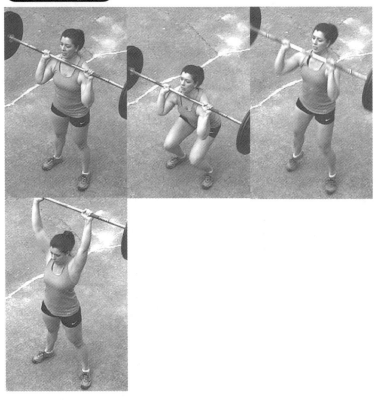

- Place your O-bar on the rack at chest level.
- Step under the bar and place it in clean position.
- Hit a quarter squat and then with a quick burst with the legs send the bar to a locked position overhead.
- Keeping that back tight throughout is a must.

Push-ups

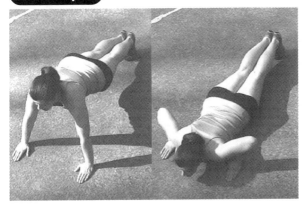

● Place your hands on the floor, palms underneath shoulders, body held in a strict plank, feet together, balls of the feet on the floor.

● Keep your head up and looking forward away from the floor throughout, descend until your chest and upper thighs brush the floor.

● Return to the locked-out position.

Side bar
"But I can't do push-ups!"

No sweat. This is an easy one to build quickly, far easier than building your dips and pull-ups. The following points helped me:

● I keep my core tight and my shoulders pinched throughout allowing the body to sag seems to sap strength.

● I also think of tucking my elbows in toward my sides as I push back to lock out. *Continued next page.*

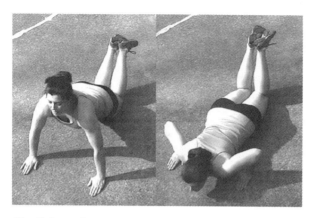

Partial push-up

If that doesn't work, start with the so-called "girl push-up" which begins from the knees as opposed to the balls of the feet.

Just keep all of the standard push-up tips in mind and keep your eyes on the prize of being able to do the real thing so you we can make that the New Girl Push-Up!

Rope pull-ups

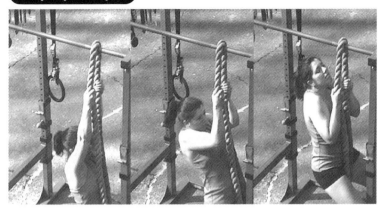

Rope climb or rope pull-ups

A length of 15 foot climbing rope is ideal, but some of us may not have a place to hang one in a home gym. Anytime you see a rope climb posted in a daily challenge, substitute 10 rope pull-ups per prescribed climb.

● For a rope pull-up, throw your rope over your pull-up bar.
● Grip the rope with both hands and from a dead-hang pull until your chin is even with your fists.

Rope shinny

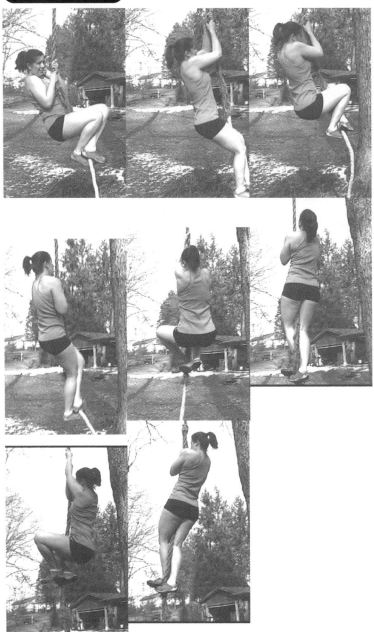

If you have access to a fixed climbing rope:

● Reach as high as you can and grip the rope with both hands.
● Tuck your legs toward your chest allowing the rope to pass between your legs.
● Use a squeeze between the outside blades of your feet to gain a purchase on the rope.
● Reach one hand and then the other as high as you are comfortable and repeat the process.

Shin to chin (S2C)

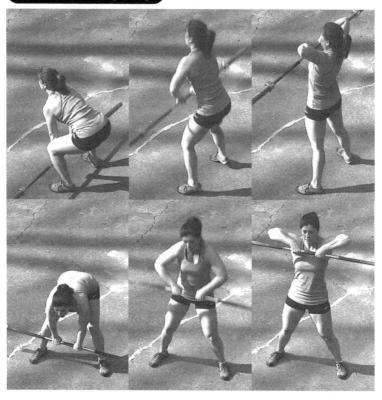

● Shin to chins (S2C from here on out) are an endurance exercise.

● Lay an unloaded O-bar on the ground.

● Take a stance slightly wider than shoulder's width.

● Grip the bar with your hands approximately 6-8 inches apart.

● From a quarter squat position with head up and back flat, stand upright and surge the bar toward your chin until your upper arms are parallel with your shoulders.

● Repeat this process with the bar always travelling this approximate upper shin level to chin level.

● A big mistake is to not use the quarter squat on each rep and simply bend forward at the waist That's half an exercise — don't waste your time.

Sprint

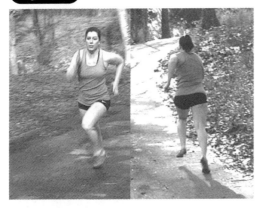

● Exactly what it sounds like — an all-out run as fast as you can for the designated distance.

Squats

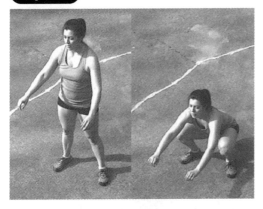

● Same mechanics as the prisoner squat but here you don't lock your hands behind your head.
● You can swing them in any manner that you see fit to improve your rate of speed.

Squat ball

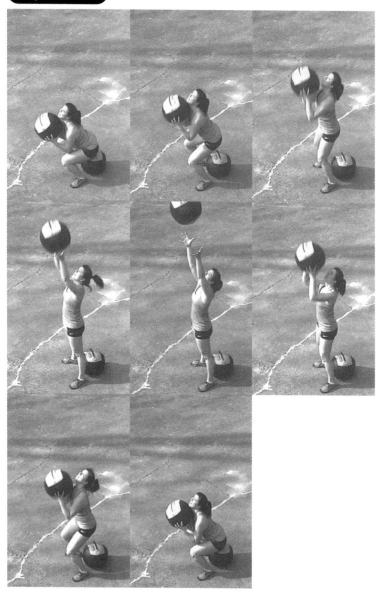

- This is a variant of an exercise commonly known as wall ball.
- Place your butt-bumper on the ground, hold another 20# medicine ball at clean position.
- Squat to the bumper and as you come to your full stand toss the ball into the air above you approximately 1-2 feet (or more).
- Catch the ball and repeat.

Squat clean

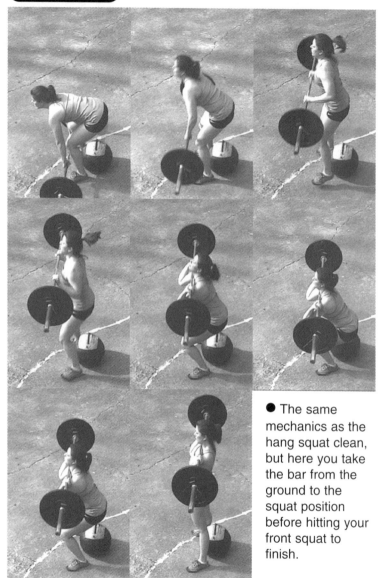

● The same mechanics as the hang squat clean, but here you take the bar from the ground to the squat position before hitting your front squat to finish.

Strict press

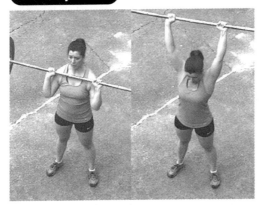

● A variant of the push press with no leg assist.
● Rack your O-bar at shoulder level and step under it.
● With the bar in clean position and using no assist from the legs, press the bar to an overhead locked position.
● I find that it helps to pinch my shoulders, lock my back and tighten my butt before I press.

Sweep backs or GHD sit-ups

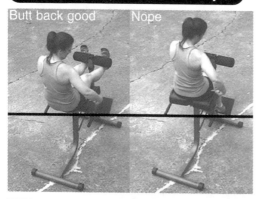

Butt back good   Nope

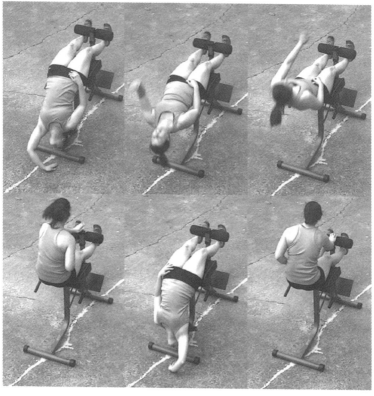

● A tough one for the entire front of the body: abdominals, hip flexors, and quadriceps.

● Sit on the stand and lock your ankles under the foot catch.

● Slide your butt off the stand so that only your upper hamstrings are on the stand — your body will stay in this perch throughout the exercise.

● Lean backward until you can brush the deck with your fingertips.

● Fling your arm forward until you come to a 90 degree bend and touch your knee with your hand.

Terrain run

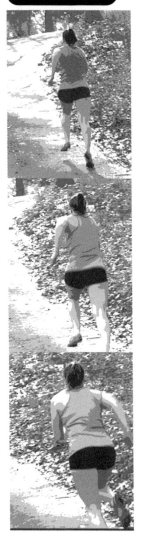

● Anytime a run is prescribed either as a "designated distance" or simply "Cover as much distance as you can in a designated time," ideally you will make these runs along off-road running trails. The more variety in terrain the better, that is, hills to climb and go down, rocks and stumps to navigate and so on.

● Failing an off-road trail, find an urban trail that provides as much stimulus as you can safely manage: curbs to hop, a low wall to go over, uneven surfaces to navigate, that sort of thing.

● What I want to urge you away from is flat tracks, smooth, paved running trails and anything that makes our run "easier." (God forbid, you do these on a treadmill. Don't be a hamster.)

● I'd rather see you running around your backyard jumping over the kid's toys than taking one of these smoother options.

Thrusters

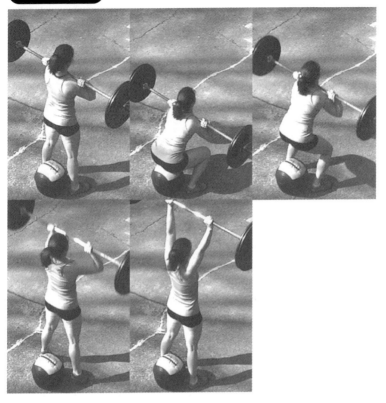

- This is a combination exercise that will really get the body hating you.
- It is simply a front squat combined with a push press.
- Set your butt-bumper.
- Clean the bar and drop to a front squat.
- Stand and hit your push press.
- That's one rep. Enjoy!

Toes to bar

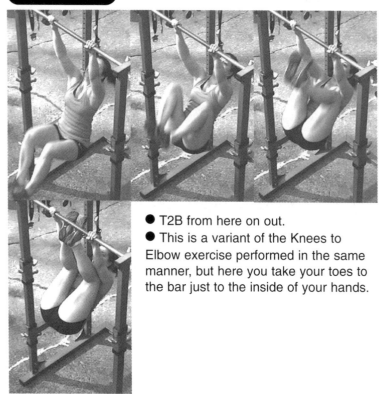

- T2B from here on out.
- This is a variant of the Knees to Elbow exercise performed in the same manner, but here you take your toes to the bar just to the inside of your hands.

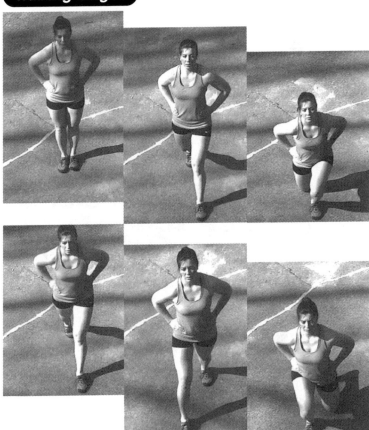

- With your hands on your hips, take one long step forward with your left foot until your left knee is just kissing the ground.
- Repeat with the right leg. - Stay upright and your back straight. Not leaning forward will keep you from overloading that lead leg excessively.

Good and bad posture.

Walking lunges with weight plate

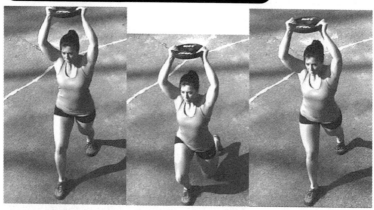

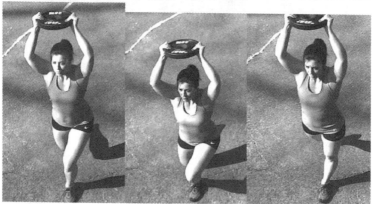

● Same as the walking lunge, but here you have the fun of holding a plate in locked out position while you hit your lunges.

Weighted pull-ups

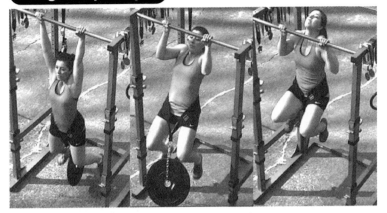

● Exactly what it sounds like. Use a weight belt or hold a dumbbell between your feet and you'll be good to go.

For additional exercises and video tutorials on many of these and more, see my website at www.cosmonot.us

She's Tough

7. Menus

Here are your 60 completely different daily challenges

They are meant to be hit in order and not in a mix and match manner. You can mix and match if you want to, but I find that mixing and matching leads to cherry-picking, that is, giving short shrift to the truly tough days and emphasizing the easier ones.

At the end of workout 60, you can start though the sequence again to chart your improvement, or head over to my site for access to brand spanking new challenges: www.cosmonot.us

How often to train is your call. Me? I do three days on and one day off 52 weeks a year barring illness or holidays.

You might be more comfortable with a three days a week or every other day schedule. The point is, find a schedule that works for you and stick to it; we'll never get to Texas if we manufacture pit stops left and right.

1.
Bench press @ BW (25/50/75) 10
Pull-ups 10
Countdown both

2.
Shin to chin w/O-bar (200/150/100)

3.
Burpees (100/75/50)

4.
Dumbbell (DB) ground to overhead (30/20/10) 100
Use two DBs and get both to an overhead proof of lift, touching the ground with both DBs at the bottom of each repetition.

5.
Pull-up/toes to bar combo (50/40/25)
Hit a pull-up and at the bottom of a dead hang hit a toes to bar rep. That's one rep.

6.
Walking lunge with weight plate
(25/10/broomstick overhead)
300 yards

7.
100-yard sprint
Xs 10/8/6
Rest 45 seconds between efforts.

8.
Overhead squats (95/75/45) 10
Low hurdle hops 50/40/30
Xs 3

9.
Deadlift (185/155/135) 100/75/50

10.
Overhead squat (95/75/45) 75/50/30

11.
Thrusters (75/65/45) 100/75/50

12.
Pull-up fatigue 50/30/25
Each time you come off the bar, hit a 20-yard shuttle run and get back on the bar immediately.

Side bar
"What is a shuttle run?"

● Place two cones or markers 10 yards apart.
● Sprint to the far cone, bend and touch the line.
● Sprint back to the first cone.
● All of the above is expected to be performed as quickly and explosively as possible.

13.
Back squat
5 singles to find your 1RM

14.
Terrain run (3 miles/2 miles/1 mile)

15.
Back pedal (half mile/quarter mile/200 yards)

16.
Deadlift
5 singles to your 1RM

17.
Run 1/4 Mile
Overhead kettlebell (KB) swing (45/35/25) 50/30/20
Xs 3

18.
Run 1/4 Mile
Pull-ups 25/15/10
Xs 3

19.
Sprint 100 Yards
Deadlift (225/185/135) 1
Xs 10

20.
Death by pull-ups
1 rep on minute 1
2 in minute 2
Continue until you tap.

21.
Death by dips
Rings for the pros and bar dips for the rookies.

22.
Box jumps (24/20/18 inches) (150/100/75)

23.
Leaping pull-ups 75/50/25
Place a mark 3 feet from the bar. Leap from the mark to the bar and complete your pull-up off of the initial swing. Come off the bar and return to the mark.

24.
Overhead KB swings (45/35/25) 150/100/75

25.
Walking lunges
1/2 mile for pros/1/4 mile for intermediate/200 yards for rookies.

26.
Knees to elbows fatigue 100/50/25
Each time you come off the bar, hit a 20-yard shuttle run and get back on the bar immediately.

27.
O-bar thruster fatigue (100/75/50)
Use an empty O-bar. Each time you have to rest hit a 20-yard shuttle run and hit the bar immediately.

28.
Burpees
Low hurdle hops
50/40/30/20/10
30/20/10
20/15/10

29.
Deadlift (225/185/135) 3
Prisoner squats 10/8/6
Xs 10

30.
Overhead squat (95/75/45) 3
Push-ups 10/8/6
Xs 10

31.
Death by pull-ups
1 rep in minute 1
2 in minute 2
Continue until you can't fit the work inside the minute.

32.
Death by dips
Rings for pros, bar for rookies.

33.
Terrain run (3 miles/2 miles/1 mile)

34.
Front squat (155/135/95) 5
Run 1/4 mile
Xs 4

35.
Pull-ups 10/8/6
Sprint 100 Yards
Xs 10

36.
Overhead KB swing (45/35/25) 25/20/15
Run 1/4 mile
Xs 4

37.
Squat ball 250/175/100

38.
Bench press (95/75/55) 10
Sprint 100 yards
Xs 10

39.
Terrain run (3 miles/2 miles/1 mile)

40.
Back squat
5 sets of 2 to find your 2RM

41.
Overhead KB swing (40/30/30) 10
Pull-ups 10
Countdown both (elbow hitch pull-ups for the pros)

42.
Shin to chins 250/150/75

43.
Thrusters (75/65/55) 5
Hang power cleans (75/65/55) 10
Rounds in 20 minutes

44.
Sprint 100 yards
Xs 10/8/6
Rest 90 seconds between

45.
Run 1 mile/ .5 miles/ .25 miles
Back squat (95/75/55) 50
Repeat the run
Bench press (95/75/55) 50
Repeat the run

46.
Push press
5 singles to your 1RM

47.
Hang squat clean
Five 2s to your 2RM

48.
Maximum number of push-ups in 15 minutes

49.
Maximum number of squats in 15 minutes

50.
Deadlift (185/155/135) 5
Low hurdle hops 50/30/20
Xs 5

51.
Maximum number of burpees in 12 minutes

52.
Power clean (95/85/75) 10
Dips 10
Countdown both

53.
Terrain run
Maximum distance covered in 30 minutes

54.
Grab a single dumbbell (40/30/20) and take it for a 1.5 mile terrain walk.

55.
Back squat
Five 5s to find your 5RM

56.
Sprint 100 yards
Prisoner squats 50/30/20
Xs 5

57.
Toes to bar 10
Thrusters (95/75/55) 10
Countdown both

58.
Shoulder press
Five 1s to find your 1RM

59.
Pull-ups 5 (strict pull-ups for you pros)
Box jumps (24"/20"/18") 8
Overhead KB swing (40/30/20) 10
Xs 10

60.
Clean & jerk (95/75/55) 50/30/20

You're at the end of the 60

Now it's decision time. You can either repeat the
sequence to check yourself against your benchmarks
for improvement or head over to my site www.cos-
monot.us for brand new challenges to keep you motivated.

8. Post Workout Flexibility / Mobility

Just in case you were wondering, "Don't I need to stretch out before I workout?" No, definitely not.

As a matter of fact, the science is dead set against it. For the scientific skinny, refer to the resources I mentioned in the "Yeah, but..." section.

But there is some convincing data that shows that a little post-workout flexibility or mobility work can be of value. Keep in mind, the data is a little all over the place on this one, so don't feel that if you are skipping the stretching/flexibility/mobility work that you are cheating yourself. This is sort of a cool down bonus if you have the time and feel like doing it.

You can run your own routine or none at all. Below I offer the six I use that were originally offered by Brian Mackenzie in the pages of *Outside* magazine. I've long forgotten the names of them (if they even had official names), so apologies to Mr. Mackenzie for that. Instead you'll have to suffer through what I call them.

Hip popper

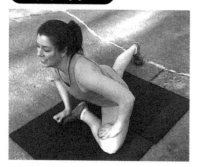

● Have a seat on the floor with your right leg before you lying on its side — the knee at an approximate 90 degree bend.
● Despite appearances, you will not sit back on your butt and simply bend forward, instead …
● Keep your butt off of the floor and your back straight. Lean forward as you think about pushing your hip (still held off of the floor) 45 degrees and backward toward your rear pocket.
● We are striving to feel this one throughout our hip and lower back region.
● Repeat on the opposite side.

Half arch

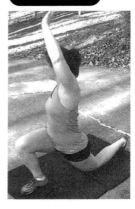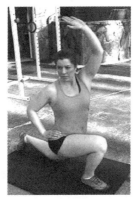

● Squat and place your left knee well behind you as you step forward and down on your right foot.

● Keeping your torso upright, drive forward toward your right foot as you get a good stretch across your hip flexor.

● You can add a little stink to this one by reaching the left arm up as you give a little turn toward your right.

● Repeat on the other side.

Bent Achilles tendon stretch

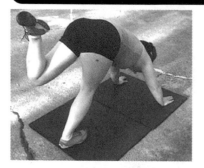

● I find that this one after long runs or heavy lifting days does the job for keeping my lower legs loose.
● Keeping the right foot flat on the ground and the knee bent (not straight) work around until you can feel a good stretch throughout that tendon.
● Repeat on the opposite side.

Squat

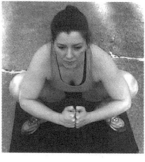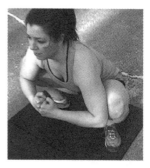

● An easy one that does wonders for the lower back.
● Keeping your feet flat, squat as low as you can go.
● Sit here, hang out and rock around a little bit to loosen the legs, hips and back.

Couch stretch

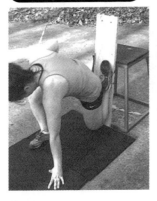 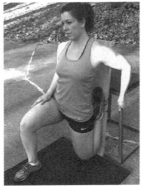

● Place your right instep and shin against an upright surface.
● With the sole of the left foot on the ground, strive to drive backward while keeping your body upright for a nicely intense stretch.
● Don't mistake a harsh curve in your back for being upright and back straight. Only lean back as far as you can with good form.
● Repeat on the other side.

Shoulder hang

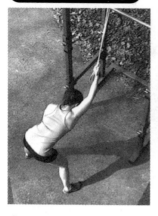
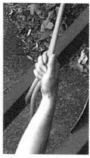
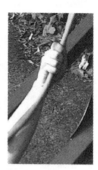

Proper grip   Not

● After a shoulder injury, this one got me back on the right path.

● Throw a stretch band or towel over a pull-up bar or even an open door.

● Grip the band and turn your palm upward — you will keep your palm upward throughout.

● Lean down and away from whatever is anchoring your band and work on loosening that shoulder.

Again, don't feel that you have to do these, but I find that these six keep me prepared for the next day's challenge.

Happy Trails

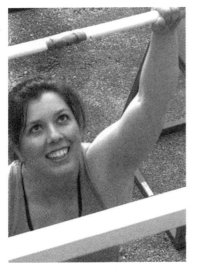

Well, here we are at the end of the trail. Have we made it to Texas yet? Probably not. This is no reflection on you — I say probably not meaning that none of us have got to where we want to be yet as this fitness journey is a long and continuous one.

Yes, we can and will have benchmarks and triumphs to celebrate all along the way, but this is one journey that isn't supposed to stop. We're meant to keep moving until our final days. Sure, we all slow down as we near the end, but there's no reason not to hold off that slowdown as long as we can and to make our "slow" seem not so slow in the end.

I hope you've got something out of the information in this book, and I would absolutely love to hear about your progress.

If you have any questions, please don't hesitate to contact me via my site www.cosmonot.us or by e-mail at kylie@cosmonot.us

But don't stop there. If you've made progress (and I don't care how much or little you think it is) let me know about it. I want you to get the most out of this journey. You may not believe me, but if you read this book and get up and do something, anything to get going to Texas, I'll be your biggest fan.

Let me hear about it and I will cheer you on. One more time with the Texas Proverb:

> Cowards never started
> The weak never got here
> & the unfit don't stay

Happy Trails, Ladies, let's show them all what we're made of!

Kylie Hatmaker, 2014

Resources

www.cosmonot.us
My site, as you well know by now. Here you'll find further challenges, support articles, and some motivation — Texas-style, of course.

www.walmart.com
For your basic gear needs (Olympic bar, plates, kettlebells, et ctera) it's hard to beat these prices.

www.dickssportinggoods.com
Another good gear supplier.

www.powersystems.com
A good supplier for some of your harder to find gear needs (bumper plates and the like). Can be pricey, but the gear is of good quality.

And, I would be a little remiss and less than grateful if I didn't mention the sites and further work of the two men who assisted with this project (they're tough in their own way).

www.startupsports.com
This is Doug Werner's site (the publisher of this book). Check it out for other great fitness titles.

www.extremeselfprotection.com
My husband, Mark Hatmaker's site. If you have an interest in MMA or reality street self-defense, give it a look.

She's Tough

Index

Books by Mark Hatmaker

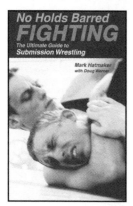

**No Holds Barred Fighting:
The Ultimate Guide
to Submission Wrestling**
The combat art of The Ultimate Fighting
Championships.
978-1-884654-17-6 / $12.95
695 photos

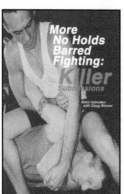

**More No Holds Barred Fighting:
Killer Submissions**
More takedowns, rides and submissions
from the authors of *No Holds Barred
Fighting.*
978-1-884654-18-3 / $12.95
650 photos

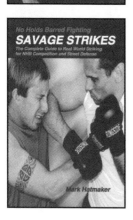

**No Holds Barred Fighting:
Savage Strikes**
*The Complete Guide to Real World
Striking for NHB Competition
and Street Defense*
Punches, kicks, forearm shots, head
butts and more.
978-1-884654-20-6 / $12.95
850 photos

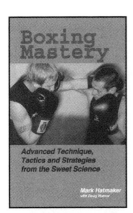

Boxing Mastery
Advance Techniques, Tactics and Strategies from the Sweet Science
Advanced boxing skills and ring generalship.
978-1-884654-29-9 / $12.95
900 photos

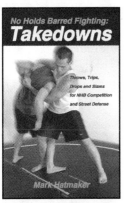

No Holds Barred Fighting: Takedowns
Throws, Trips, Drops and Slams for NHB Competition and Street Defense
978-1-884654-25-1 / $12.95
850 photos

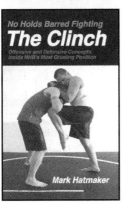

No Holds Barred Fighting: The Clinch
Offensive and Defensive Concepts Inside NHB's Most Grueling Position
978-1-884654-27-5 / $12.95
750 photos

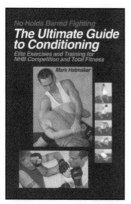

No Holds Barred Fighting:
The Ultimate Guide to Conditioning
Elite Exercises and Training for NHB
Competition and Total Fitness
978-1-884654-29-9 / $12.95
900 photos

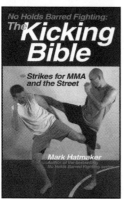

No Holds Barred Fighting:
The Kicking Bible
Strikes for MMA and the Street
978-1-884654-31-2 / $12.95
700 photos

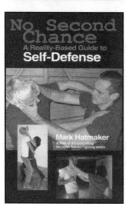

No Second Chance:
A Reality-Based Guide to Self-Defense
How to avoid and survive an assault.
978-1-884654-32-9 / $12.95
500 photos

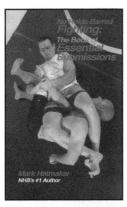

**No Holds Barred Fighting:
The Book of Essential Submissions**
How MMA champions gain their victories. A catalog of winning submissions.
978-1-884654-33-6 / $12.95
750 photos

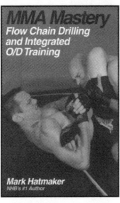

**MMA Mastery: Flow Chain Drilling
and Integrated O/D Training
to Submission Wrestling**
Blends all aspects of the MMA fight game into devastating performances.
978-1-884654-38-1 / $13.95
800 photos

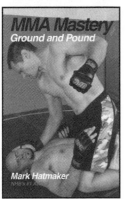

MMA Mastery: Ground and Pound
A comprehensive go-to guide — how to win on the ground.
978-1-884654-39-8 / $13.95
650 photos

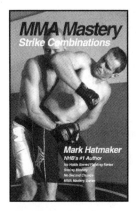

MMA Mastery: Strike Combinations
Learn the savage efficiency of striking in combinations. A comprehensive guide.
978-1-935937-22-7 / $12.95
1,000 photos

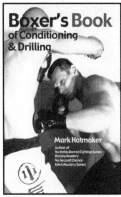

**Boxer's Book of
Conditioning & Drilling**
How to get fighting fit like the champions.
978-1-935937-28-9 / $12.95
650 photos

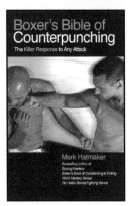

Boxer's Bible of Counterpunching
The Killer Response to Any Attack
978-1-935937-47-0 / $12.95
500 photos